Overcoming *an* ANGRY VAGINA

Journey to Womb Wellness

Queen Afua

Overcoming An Angry Vagina: Journey to Womb Wellness

The author gratefully acknowledges permission to use
illustrations and photographs by the following individuals.
Illustration & Photography
Sacred Gather of Wombmen Photos © Robert Gay
Front Cover Art: Mshundo I
Cover & Text Design: Camden Leeds, www.printnetinc.com
Text Design, Layout, Graphs & Charts: Cindy Shaw, www.printnetinc.com
Developmental Editor: Gerianne Scott
Contributing Researchers: Autumn Marie, Mitzi Bryan, Gerianne Scott

Afrikan World Books
2217 Pennsylvania Ave
Baltimore, MD 21217
410-383-2006
www.afrikanworldbooks.com

ISBN: 978-0-9779175-2-5

First Edition – Black Ankh Publications – GB – March, 2010
Revised Edition – Afrikan World Books – US – July, 2010

WOMB AWAKENING

I have awakened to Womb Wisdom.
I have stretched my heart and my soul to the universe,
crying out for a womb healing...
my prayer has been answered;
my consciousness has awakened, so I bless in advance
the rebirth of my Lotus-like womb.
As I journey deep inside myself to discover the secret healing
of the Lotus; I find a seed, the Lotus seed of illumination
that so sweetly dwells in the mist of the mud, within me.
This is a place where my lessons and trials reside.
This is the beginning of my womb healing;
my womb awakening.

Queen Afua

Table of Contents

PORTAL ONE – GUIDE TO WOMB WELLNESS

PORTAL TWO – STORIES

PORTAL THREE – STORM BEFORE THE CALM

PORTAL FOUR – REBIRTH OF WOMB WELLNESS

PORTAL FIVE – CELEBRATION

Dedication

$\mathcal{W}$ith the Womb of my Mind, the Womb of my Heart and the Womb of my Sacred
Seat, **I dedicate** *Overcoming an Angry Vagina: Journey to Womb Wellness*

...to women from the four directions East, West, North and South—
alone; in a relationship; satisfied; struggling, blissful...

...to happy, vibrant, luscious, joyous, wombs.

...to sensitive, supportive, loving partners of women who have angry vaginas.

...to unborn babies that they may be born of parents who have overcome
the negativity of an angry vagina or a hostile penis.

...to those who suffer from broken, hurt and unresolved womb trauma.

...to Wombs and Souls who cry out, "No more; No more suffering."

...to an anonymous little girl who had an abortion at age eleven.

...to a young sister who contracted womb cancer at age sixteen as her mother
stood by filled with anxiety about how to help the child of her womb.

...to the woman who frantically informed me of her fourth miscarriage. She
had lost four babies; each in her fourth month of pregnancy.

...to the many women in quest of hysterectomy prevention.

...to women who have had a hysterectomy and are ready to reclaim the
spirit of their womb.

...to women and men who suffer from the AIDS virus and STDs.

...to my daughter and my granddaughters and my sons and my grandsons

...to a new world reaching for change.

I dedicate *Overcoming an Angry Vagina: Journey to Womb Wellness* to women on an
inner quest for new womb stories and lives of rebirth, hope, love, forgiveness, enlightenment, restoration, empowerment...and to the men who love and honor these
women, as they love and honor themselves.

May we purify and rejuvenate. May we collectively take our wombs, our destiny and
our lives, into our own hands and birth a world of peace and harmony.

I dedicate this text to you. With all my heart,

Queen Afua

I Am The Angry Vagina

Most of the time, I have a happy, joyous, moist, energized vagina. But, on occasion I have a stressed out, hurt, lonely and angry vagina.

Yes, I have an attitude! I am the Angry Vagina. Like a time capsule all of life has-been absorbed into and through my vagina.

Hemorrhaging! 7, 10, 14 days a month. The doctor calls my flow "normal." The doctor says my agonizing suffering, bedridden clotting and pain are "normal." I have been cursed, like all women. Yes, I have an attitude!

As a young woman, I became a sexual addict, jumping from man to man; searching for comfort in the bed with whomever I thought would give me what I was missing in my heart. Hopeless, I end with more pain and more emptiness... Yes, I have an attitude! I am the Angry Vagina.

Meanwhile, despite the pain and drama of having my period, I'm glad to see it. I breathe a sigh of relief, I'm not pregnant. That guy was a loser. I don't want a loser to be my baby's father. Yes, I have an attitude! I am the Angry Vagina.

I'm on my third abortion today. I create. I destroy. I've got an attitude about my life choices. My vagina is angry!

Incest as far back as I can remember with father, uncle, cousin, brother...Mother passing me around like a food platter. Yes, I have an attitude! I am the Angry Vagina.

I dreamed of being married, wanted a sense of love and security by any means. Then it happened. I became the good wife; my husband took care of me. To pay him back whenever he wanted sex and I did not, I just laid there counting spots on the ceiling. I numbed my feelings, left my body for him to do his business, over and over again. My pleasure did not matter. Yes, I have an attitude. I am the Angry Vagina.

Go away, fibroid tumors, growing in me like parasite monsters feeding off my life force. I always wanted to have a baby; conceiving was difficult. When I finally got pregnant, you, tumors, were still in my womb. In the 16th week of my pregnancy, you, tumors, won my womb space and pushed out my baby...and then a second time and again a third time....Yes, I am the Angry Vagina.

I got pregnant, went full term, developed toxemia so I had to have a C-section or lose life, mine or the baby's. They cut me in half, surgically. I want my baby and I want to live. Is this my only choice? Yes, I have an attitude! I am the Angry Vagina.

I was faithful to my husband and still I contracted an STD. How could this happen to me? Yes, I have an attitude! I am the Angry Vagina.

I had fibroid tumors removed in my 20's but they grew back again in my 30's. To add insult to injury, now I have been diagnosed with abnormal cells..."down there." I was told to get a hysterectomy and then all my problems would disappear. No! My girlfriends, mother, and aunt all had hysterectomies and they still got problems. Yes, we have attitudes! We are the Angry Vaginas.

I am a menopausal woman. It should be my time of maturity to enjoy being a wise woman. Instead I am in menopausal shock! My womb is dried up and prolapsed; dropping out. My bones are brittle. My spirit is drained. Yes, I have an attitude! I am the Angry Vagina.

Into a circle of women, I was carried, limp, hurt, saddened, disheartened, angry. They asked me what I felt. My vagina spoke up for me and said we feel numb, confused. Then she said, "We are angry!" My vagina screamed a primal scream that echoed in the womb of my heart and the womb of my soul and stopped my world on its axis. Then she wept and told her story and cried a river of tears that healed us.

I can see my way home. I begin to take my journey to womb recovery. I begin to take back my power. The Womb of my Mind begin to think and create. The Womb of my Heart begins to feel reborn and renewed. Each day I come out of the mud washing layers off myself. My soul is rejuvenating away from the rage.

I have vision, hope and purpose, even though others have told me it is impossible; it's only a dream. I keep right on living to birth my purpose. Even when there is no more water for my garden to grow and my vision seems about to die, I continue on my path of rebirth. Hopelessness and anger are leaving. I will give birth to a liberated peace-filled, radiantly vibrant life. The sun is rising through me. Sunlight is shining through me. I am reclaiming the healer within me. I am free to birth a world of wellness.

Editor's Preface

NOT YOUR MAMA'S METAPHOR

*O*vercoming an Angry Vagina: Journey to Womb Wellness, a self-help guide for balance and empowerment is a book for all humans. The focus of the text is the womb –the first cradle for every human infant; and the vagina –the womb's pathway and sentinel.

The vagina is also known as, "yoni", "seshet", "sacred seat", "khat", "pussy", "coochie", "snatch", "la-la", poo-nan-nie", "va-jay-jay", "cookie", "cho-cho", "pum-pum", "purse" *and* "pocket-book", "cunt" and "possible." (Grandma used to say, "Wash up as far as possible, then wash down as far as possible, then wash possible!")

The vagina is outraged about global atrocities committed against women and their wombs. Whether lifted by Cesarean (C-section) or delivered by vaginal birth, even embryos "planted" by in vitro fertilization—every human is born from the womb. It is time to examine the impact of the atrocities on wombs in particular and on global wellness in general.

Hysterectomies are "routine." Clitoridectomies are as brutal as crime scenes. Rape, abuse and misinformation are among the acts that jeopardize women's minds, bodies, spirits and/or experiences. These acts are performed in the name of religion, medicine, legislation and/or even LOVE. They are sanctioned by men *and women* and accepted as "That's the way it is." Wombs have been damaged. The wellness of all humans has been damaged. Womb wellness must become a global concern. Overcoming an angry vagina is a global urgency.

Herein, **"an angry vagina"** is a provocative metaphor for global outrage against damage to wombs. At some point in her life, every woman **has, will have,** or—

best case scenario—*has had* an angry vagina. **"Not me,"** you say? Statistical evidence inclusive of all demographics says that womb damage exists regardless of wealth, ethnicity, sexual orientation, religious expression, political affiliation, dietary habits and/or geographic location. Because the commissions and/or omissions of **any** of us have an impact on **all** of us, damaged wombs were/are present in the bedroom and in the boardroom and in the bush. They were/are present in each victim *and* each perpetrator of **all holocausts.** Mothers, daughters, brides and entrepreneurs, prisoners, scientists and divas have wounded wombs. So do wives, activists, sisters and artists. The presence of angry vaginas anywhere announces the existence of worldwide womb crisis.

According to ancient Nile Valley text, the lotus seed emerges from the mud as a vibrant blossom. Herein, **"overcoming the angry"** is the metaphor for becoming "unstuck" from the mud of life's challenges. The overcoming, the "blooming", is an ongoing evolution of consciously and actively "healing thyself."

Many world religions profess that when a woman disobeyed God; humanity was cursed. Their doctrines validate the pain and suffering of childbirth and menstruation (often called "the curse") as manifestations of Divine wrath.

Commandments and civil laws were written as prophylactics against female sinfulness. Customs and taboos further disarmed women. Metaphorically and actually, women were placed on pedestals and/or tethered to men's leashes. This simultaneous invention of virgins and whores reduced women to objects and property. Physically, mentally, emotionally, economically, spiritually and culturally women were *un-empowered.* Predictably, imbalances on every level caused cycles of systemic *dis*-eases. Broken hearts, broken homes, damaged minds and damaged wombs can be traced to disease-causing thoughts, emotions and acts. Few humans are immune to the imbalance and the anger.

Historically, those who attempted to break the cycle with unsanctioned rituals were called *witches.* They were prosecuted, stoned, burned at the stake. Currently, those who *dare* to defy convention with gestures of self-definition are called *bitches.* Their access to food, housing, health-care, education and employment is compromised. Psychological and financial disenfranchisement is no more "civilized" than burning and stoning, as some might argue. Horrifically, archaic tortures continue to be practiced throughout the world. Pedestals—and the women on them—become more gilded; shabby tethers tighten women into shabbier conditions. Wombs are under attack by laws etched in stone. Overcoming an angry vagina is about breaking these laws of imbalance.

The text of **Overcoming an Angry Vagina: Journey to Womb Wellness** is divided into five portals (doorways). **PORTAL ONE: Guide to Global Womb Wellness** offers physical, mental, emotional and spiritual strategies for restoring empowerment, balance and wellness. In **PORTAL TWO: Stories** stand on Common Ground. They whisper and scream our lives. **PORTAL THREE: Storm Before the Calm** is a global timeline of womb damage. **PORTAL FOUR: Rebirth** encourages realizing self and visions. **PORTAL FIVE: Celebration** presents poses of the Dance of the Womb and Womb Yoga for celebration of liberation and wellness.

Queen Afua, a wholistic practitioner for over thirty-two years, has examined the intrinsic relationship between the state of the womb and the level of wellness. She passionately assures us that we can heal our wombs, our families and our world. She advocates that each woman's priority must be her own womb wellness. Remember, "If Mama ain't happy, ain't nobody happy." We must heal our thoughts and emotions in order to heal our actions and relationships. Queen Afua is confident that as womb wellness becomes a global priority and women and men become equally respected and accountable, we can overcome imbalance, one angry vagina at a time. Globally, we will begin to give birth to positive thoughts, responsible acts and well children.

G. F. Scott, Midnight Literary Midwife

Introduction

ANGRY VAGINAS SOS

I was inspired and led to write **Overcoming an Angry Vagina: Journey to Womb Wellness** because there is a global urgency to restore Womb Wellness. For over three decades, 95% of the women that I have counseled, guided and taught in wholistic workshops and seminars were challenged by imbalances and disharmony within their wombs. I began searching for the root cause of their conditions. I wondered why—more often than not—no matter the religious practice, the economic status, the race or the creed, globally, my clients complained of the same womb pains and dis-eases. Their complaints came as screams from angry vaginas.

Suddenly, from deep within, I heard a warning from my own womb:

> *"Wake up or I'm leaving! I can't live in this house with you unless you get some of this stuff up off of me. The mates that did not work got me angry and depressed. Your client load of everybody's pain is overloading me. Lighten up your load or I'm out of here."*

Shocked, I looked around for who was speaking, but there was nobody else. I looked down at myself and realized that the voice was coming from my womb. I paid close attention and took the steps I knew...detoxify, use wholistic herbs and tonics, fast and pray, do my Womb Yoga exercises...heal myself. Soon, my womb began to speak more at ease.

Then I looked outside of myself and studied women's womb conditions in terms of their relationship to world conditions. Conclusively, I found that there was a direct correlation between the condition of wombs and the state of the world. Through consistent observations of women, families and society, it became clear that **what** and **where** we are is dialectically linked to what is happening within our womb. The wellness of all wombs is under attack. There have been thousands of attempts to "fix" the problems. However, since these attempted remedies are not personal, definitive changes in how we take care of ourselves, the damage continues to calcify. Dis-ease continues to be accepted as "normal." Our bodies, minds and sprits are not well. Consequently, we give birth to toxic people, thoughts, actions and relationships.

Giving birth to babies from of dis-eased wombs and thoughts is what keeps the human family in chaos and discord. We have been giving birth to those who create war, steal land, enslave people, suppress women's power and manipulate nature. I asked myself, "What kind of womb environment breeds and brings forth such a low and violent frequency of humanity?" Most people are born from women suffering from toxic, suppressed and enraged thoughts. Far too many women have fibroid-filled wombs, cancerous wombs, cystic wombs, mutilated wombs, raped wombs, endometrial wombs, prolapsed wombs, abortive wombs filled with sorrow, hurt wombs, sad wombs, depressed wombs, racist wombs; have lost their wombs.

The overwhelming screams from angry vaginas are fibroid tumors. Usually noncancerous, fibroid tumors are age-old and worldwide. Other "screams" include painful menstrual cycles, infertility, abortions (legality, depends on place, time and government), difficult birthing episodes, miscarriages, troublesome menopause experiences, cancerous tumors. Eating disorders that range from obesity to anorexia announce the presence of an angry vagina. Depression, diabetes, high blood pressure, migraine headaches, STDs and vaginitis warn us that wombs are not well. Angry vaginas are screaming, "No more secrets! No more damage! No more crimes! No more wars!"

Overcoming an Angry Vagina: Journey to Womb Wellness is an invitation to pay wholistic attention to your physical, mental, emotional and spiritual and even economic wellness. It is a guide to using your nutrition habits, detoxification routines, physical exercises, prayers, meditations and spiritual activities to Heal Thyself. It is time to eliminate preventable illness and suffering. The Angry Vagina is a planetary problem. Overcoming the Angry Vagina must become a planetary priority. I encourage the reader to use the text of this volume, as well as strategies provided in my previous works, to know yourself better and to empower yourself. Become a Womb Worker who heals yourself and joins others who seek to change the disharmony and overcome the anger.

Imbalance has had its hand on the power button. It is the reason why our bodies, thoughts, emotions and relationships are not as well as they should be and could be. The purpose of this text is to ignite a reversal of power and a restoration of balance. Overcoming an angry vagina is a bold step in rerouting the planet from a toxicity back to natural wholesomeness.

The strategies in this text are intended to initiate an end to disharmony and imbalance. Imbalanced thoughts have led to imbalanced emotions and imbalanced deeds. Wars have been waged. There is rampant and epidemic occurrence of dis-eases all over the planet. Overcoming an angry vagina is intended to end the blatant dishonoring of women (by men and by women) and to the restore balance, respect and honor among women and men. It is meant to inspire mutual, harmonious leadership.

A new world must begin from the restoration of Wholistically Well Wombs. Women must rise up and begin to heal themselves. Our own womb wellness must become our priority. As we heal ourselves, we become empowered. Cultivating Womb Workers to overcome angry vaginas and work toward Global Wellness is restoring humanity to wholeness, harmony and beauty. Balance...as it was in the beginning.

Queen Afua

Two Letters

– LETTER ONE –

Dear Imbalance: (Yes, **"Dear"**—for we will not curse *you* as you have cursed *us*. We simply will get rid of you!)

*F*or centuries you have been manipulating, enslaving and messing with me and my womb, my seat of creation; my symbol of "womanness." You've been suppressing, abusing and mutilating my womb in every way. I even have supported you in my own demise. My womb has been a "cash cow" for society, making big profits off my ignorance for everything from prostitution to hysterectomies. In antiquity, thousands of years before Imbalance took over, women were respected, honored and lifted up. There was harmony.

Things changed. Some religions promoted that women caused humanity to become cursed. This supported a course of action taken by men to control and suppress women on all levels. Laws were created to protect society from women's thoughts and deeds; women must blindly follow the leadership of men.

The doctrines suggested that women have to suffer with pain during their menstruation. **Not true,** Imbalance! Women who live a natural toxin-free life can have a pain-free monthly cycle with minimal bleeding of one to three days! Some beliefs claimed that women were cursed to suffer greatly during childbirth. Again, **Not true!** Women who embrace natural-living and eliminate flesh and fast foods from their diet can experience childbirth and labor reduced from the common 12 to 36 hour battle to a 2 to 6 six hour process of bearable womb contractions. When complimented with proper breathing, a woman can experience and embrace natural birthing without synthetic medication or drugs of any kind.

As a rite of passage within some cultures, young girls are raised and trained to submit willingly to clitoral castration. During the procedure, usually without anesthesia, they must suffer silently as their flesh is cut away. The pain, a customary part of these rites, is encouraged to keep these young girls "in check."

Listen, you, Imbalance – Take your hand off the power button! Your reign of illness is being defused. You've been running things for over 2000 years. You've been running us into war, violence, disharmony and tragedy. In antiquity, we lived in balance with each other and with nature. We enjoyed Wellness. It was a Golden Age.

Well, we are back! The healers in us are awakening and rebirthing themselves. We are getting back on our seat; we are using our healing tools. Yes, we women, we Angry Vaginas, we Womb Workers in our own lives, we will bring balance to the equation of our lives. We, who embrace Womb Wisdom, will return this planet to BALANCE through Womb Wellness Recovery. We are taking the steps of overcoming angry vaginas. Women of the world are speaking out and organizing against the practice of female castration that continues to this very moment. Women of the world are transforming their lives of shame, rape and incest. We are overcoming the global angry vaginas. Righteous women and men are proclaiming: It's a NEW DAY....It's a NEW TIME...It's a NEW BEGINNING!

Beware, Imbalance. BALANCE IS ON THE RISE!!

– LETTER TWO –

Dear Seekers of Balance:

Come into Womb Recovery, it is time to heal your life and birth a New World. To heal your life you must experience a rebirth. Wake up to your inner wisdom. Start from the seed of yourself (your Bloodline.). Return to the seed of thought that created your flesh and bones, the condition of your heart, your temperament, your attitude, your experiences, your relationships. Your body, mind and spiritual wombs begin as seeds in the womb surrounded by mud. As you continue your bloodlines, dare to make your own choices. Will your seeds flourish *or perish?*

Come into womb awareness. Consciously or unconsciously, your thoughts and your feelings reflect the condition of your womb. What you think and feel is what you birth. When your womb is nourished, fulfilled and purified, it births joy and bliss. If your womb is starved, abused, unappreciated or toxic, it births pain and sorrow, heavy bleeding and cramps. Your womb-state dictates whether you give birth to dis-ease or wellness in both physical and visionary forms. You are welcomed to overcome an angry womb, to rehabilitate and mend your broken life and broken heart and to give birth to your wholeness. Return to your original state of illumination on the physical and mental planes. Become instruments in creating a world of harmony that replaces a world where women suffer from heavy menstrual flow, vaginitis, cysts, fibroid tumors, STDs, PMS, prolapsed wombs, miscarriage, infertility and sexual abuse. Increase your wellness as you increase your balance. In our minds, the womb of our thoughts, we must create new thoughts. In our womb hearts we must rebirth new temperaments, attitudes, relationships. When we detoxify and properly nourish our wombs we will begin to heal ourselves.

Seek balance through the elements of air, fire, water and earth; become one with nature. When we detoxify for purification and empower ourselves with wholistic nutrition and lifestyle we can unify into a mighty force of wellness for personal and Global Healing. As Seekers of Balance, overcoming angry vaginas, become the seed, breaking through the water and mud to blossom as a full Lotus Being.

Overcome, rise above and fulfill your Destiny. Forgive, restore and begin again.

It is time to heal the people, to birth a new day, to restore planet earth. We must flush out hatred, cleanse out resentment and purge rage. We must reclaim our seat of power. We are Seekers of Balance, teaching our daughters and sons, loving our men, saving hearts and souls and saving lives. We are inspiring the birth of organic beings, who will walk in freedom. We are birthing our lives in Balance.

Seeking Balance

To all seeking balance in order to overcome an angry vagina: Use Wholistic Womb Wellness tools and strategies to address fibroid tumors, infertility, chronic PMS, menstrual and menopausal heavy bleeding and clotting, prolapsed wombs, infections and immune challenges. Global womb wellness begins with each woman's decision to restore her personal womb wellness and to overcome an angry vagina.

- Listen to the Voice of the Womb for:
  - emotional and spiritual recovery;
    - inner guidance;
      - release of womb trauma and toxic-womb drama

- Wholistically detoxify and rejuvenate
  with herbs and tonics and whole foods

- Take soothing and healing baths
  with essential oils, salts and herbs

- Offer prayers of thanksgiving and forgiveness

- Recite affirmations of redemption

- Actualize meditations of empowerment

- Guide and share in Womb Wellness Healing Circles

- Use arts and creative works to heal and restore the Inner You

- Learn and perform Womb Yoga exercises

- Learn and perform The Dance of the Womb movements

- Use Womb Wisdom to birth healthy relationships, well babies
  and vibrant visions

It's a Womb Wellness Revolution!

Prologue

Time: Friday morning, February 4th, 1994

Place: Brooklyn District Health Center

I was sitting between two dynamic medical practitioners. The distinguished Dr. Kamau Kokayi was to my left and the illustrious Dr. Josephine English was to my right. Coincidentally, Dr. English (OB/GYN) had delivered my children 18, 15, and 12 years before. Three times I entrusted her with my life and the birthing of my babies. Today, I still thank her from the depths of my womb.

The doctors and I were there to receive acknowledgement and honors from the New York City Department of Health for Women's Health services provided in the Brooklyn community. I was invited to give an acceptance speech to the community and the staff. Of course, my theme was natural methods of illness prevention and wellness strategies for reproductive health.

I believe it was on *that* Friday morning that the very first conception of Womb Wellness/Womb Wisdom was sparked. *That* Friday morning I shared my Natural Womb-Healing policy with the audience at the Department of Health. The womb of my heart was filled with the joy that soon I would be sharing my concept for developing Womb Wellness for Global Healing with a much larger audience...

Taking My Own Advice

For many years, I have been involved with the call of Liberation Thru Purification for planetary healing. Spreading the message of Heal Thyself was in my every thought. The years of persistent teaching, consulting, guiding and walking people to the Path of Purification took its toll upon me. I seemed to have reached the end of my capacity to help others, for I began to absorb the poor health conditions suffered by some of my clients and students. I desperately and absolutely needed to recharge my life, my mind, my soul, my nerves, and little did I know, my womb. February 18th, 1995 was my last day of work on this level as I received a "womb awakening."

I had been seeing 25 to 30 clients, weekly, for years. That day I had counseled eight clients –three had advanced forms of cancer and another had full-blown AIDS. I have always felt a deep compassion for every one of my clients; but had I gone beyond my ability to assist others in overcoming pain and dis-ease?

After my very last client, I experienced heaviness, a deep pulling sensation within my womb that frightened me to no end! With my palm cupped over the outside of my womb, I started to pray. I stumbled from my office into the kitchen lab where Sister Wahida was preparing Heal Thyself formulas. I told Wahida I feared for the safety of my womb; it felt like my womb was going to drop right out! As I feverishly prayed, I realized that I had experienced the aftermath of emotionally toxic womb absorption. The toxicity had to be released or my womb would be devastated. I also became aware that overwork can cause undue stress and pressure, and therefore make the womb more vulnerable to womb afflictions. I was holding my womb for dear life. Carefully I laid down on the floor and put my feet up against the wall at a 45-degree angle. I was working to prevent a prolapsed womb. The healer within me stood up and came forth to save my womb. My womb gave me step-by-step guidance on what she needed me to do to *heal*. I was guided to gently massage my womb, to breathe deeply and to pray softly.

Approximately thirty minutes later my womb began to say, "Peace!"

I wasn't feeling perfect quite yet. So, I chanted to my womb from my heart, "I love you, I love you", over and over again. "I will let you rest; I will take better care of you." With tears in my eyes, I finally said, "I will let go of my emotional baggage."

About four or five minutes later my womb was without pain. It was amazing, I felt normal again. It was during that experience that the Voice of My Womb was born. Those moments of challenge issued forth my own womb meditation, womb affirmation, Dance of the Womb and other healing steps. My own angry vagina raised her voice. I thank the Most High for both of us that I was able to listen and respond. I was one step closer to my own healing and rebirth.

(Five months later Queen went to St. Thomas for her own much-needed womb restoration. When she returned she began the first phase of this book in your hands.)

PORTAL
One

THE GUIDE
TO GLOBAL WOMB
WELLNESS

WHO, ME?

*W*omen, Sisters, Ladies: It is time for a Womb Wellness Revolution!

In this book, listen to stories told by our Sisters and Mothers and Girlfriends. Trace the timeline of global events connected to those stories.

From one portal, one doorway to the next, find your story, research your causes of dis-ease and gather your wellness tools.

Become empowered by discovering what may be blocking your wellness so that you can awaken and strengthen the "healer within."

This is a revolution, a turn-around-time to take bold, brilliant steps towards your personal wellness.

The condition of a woman's womb gives insight to what is going on within her life. Pay close attention to what your womb is saying to you; for self-knowledge becomes self-liberation. All womb traumas have root causes. Seek within to find yours. Look at your womb condition; own it so that you can begin to the work to heal yourself. Your womb is waiting for you to overcome an angry vagina. Find or create a womb circle of others who are saying, "That's enough! We want to feel better and live our lives better!" Have courage; your sisters are here with you.

The arsenal of tools and strategies in **PORTAL One** provides you with help to liberate yourself from the mental, spiritual, emotional and physical traumas that cause you drama and pain. Ask the Voice of your Womb to speak *to* you and *for* you, to help you prepare to rejuvenate.

Ask her:
"What is our trauma?"

Ask the Womb of your Mind and the Womb of your Heart:
"What is blocking our wellness?"
"What do we need to do to heal ourselves?"

When you discover the roots of what is blocking your wellness, you will be on your way to overcoming them and restoring balance. Let the Voice of your Womb help you to help yourself.

There is a direct correlation between the condition of your womb and your overall wellness. The presence of an angry vagina indicates a damaging, unwanted accumulation of suppression of old hurts in the wombs of your heart and your mind as well as waste in your reproductive womb. These accumulations of waste contribute to dis-eases in all your womb centers.

Now is the time to overcome negativity and replace it with live food nutrition, positive thoughts, and constructive, invigorating deeds. Now is the time to detox and rejuvenate.

Take charge of your life by overcoming a toxic diet and toxic lifestyle. Seek your Womb Wisdom so that eventually you can enjoy your Womb Wellness.

Come; let's get started on our Womb Wellness Revolution to overcome an angry vagina.

Fibroids – A Global Epidemic

Fibroid tumors are the overall predominant womb damage of my female clients. I have found fibroid tumors and their symptoms to be primary contributors to the existence of global angry vaginas. The screams and cries from global fibroid suffering has motivated my research into the causes of this calamity. I dedicate myself to assisting my clients in their womb wellness restoration.

With or without fibroids, my clients' complaints include: menstrual cramps, pelvic pain, heavy bleeding, clotting during menses, PMS, mood swings, vaginal itching and/or burning, vaginitis and vaginal cysts, infertility and recurrent pregnancy loss, difficult child birth and toxemia during pregnancy. Some women have some level of anemia due to the excessive and unscheduled bleeding from her womb. Some women have frequent urination or constipation because they have extra waste in their colons, which cause extra pressure on their bladder and/or rectum. A few women have shared that it is painful when they have sexual intercourse.

Globally, women are exploring methods to relieve the painful symptoms caused by these "womb invaders." Often, women are told that they should have a hysterectomy (removal of the uterus) as soon as possible. The problem with this solution is that although the fibroids are definitely gone, unfortunately, the woman's womb, her primary organ for reproduction, is also gone.

Fortunately, more women are deciding that hysterectomy is not an acceptable "cure" for getting rid of fibroids. Physically, there are hormonal changes as well as side effects to nearby organs. The loss of her womb can be as devastating to the womb of a woman's heart as it is to her body. Emotionally, the impact of losing her womb is different for each woman. These possible side effects are causing women to continue to look for alternative ways to get rid of fibroids.

Women who have access to laser myomectomy are choosing that form of surgery instead. The fibroids are removed, but the womb is not. Recovery time after myomectomy is usually about six weeks.

Fibroid Tumors the Global Grand "Damn" of Angry Vaginas

Even less invasive than myomectomy is uterine fibroid embolization (UFE). In this process, tiny particles are inserted into the fibroids to cut off blood supply and cause them to shrink. Most women who have UFE are walk-in or overnight patients and can return to normal activities in a day or two. The fibroids seem to die and the symptoms end for a while.

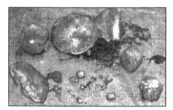

Picture of fibroid tumors in the womb

Hemorrhaging, clotting, surgery and the possible loss of the uterus: it is no wonder that women around the world have developed angry vaginas about fibroid tumors. Now we feel the need to take responsibility for the wellness of our wombs. We realize that there are always consequences to surgical procedures. We find that, whether fibroids are cut out, burned out, or "starved" out, they can *and do* grow back. We are angry and we are hurting! Now what?

Part of empowering ourselves to heal ourselves includes finding the root cause of fibroids. Usually, the origin of fibroids is omitted during treatment consultation. A woman plagued with symptoms and threatened with losing her womb is concerned with how to get rid of them. Neither she nor her physician address where these fibroids come from.

However, if she accepts the concept that, *we are what we eat,* her understanding and choices will change. Recent research reveals that fibroids have high levels of growth hormones. How are we ingesting those hormones? Are they in the air, the water, our food?

Because we can neither digest nor eliminate those hormones they remain as waste in our bodies. No wonder we have tumors! Even if we cut them out, if we eat an abundance of foods that *might* contain hormones, we invite the fibroids to return and promise to feed them.

The purpose of the strategies and tools suggested in this portal is to help you to overcome womb challenges, especially fibroid tumors. They represent over thirty years of research and practice. Fibroid tumors are benign growths found in the uterus. The size and number of fibroids usually indicates how long and how often a woman has her menses. If you detoxify the womb, you can both lessen the amount of menstrual bleeding and shrink the tumor.

Stories in this book report the experiences of women who used these detox and rejuvenating strategies to restore their womb wellness and overcome their angry vaginas. As you begin to live a Natural Lifestyle, you also will experience appropriate physical and emotional changes. You may feel sad and even find yourself crying or losing your temper. Don't be alarmed. You are cleansing. You may experience heavier menstrual bleeding for the first two months as you begin your natural cleansing (detox). Remain steadfast on your purification path. By the third or fourth month, you will begin to menstruate one-half day to one day less.

After a season of one to three months of deep cleansing, you will notice that the once solid and immobile tumor will begin to shift within your womb. Instead of being hard to touch, it will have softened. The tumor is in the process of dislodging itself; you are on your way toward womb recovery. When tumors and/or cysts soften and liquefy, the growths break up and begin draining out of your vagina. Your womb will be experiencing "natural surgery." You may have discharges or even very heavy bleeding.

It is advisable to consult your physician, especially during extreme detox symptoms (clotting, heavy bleeding, etc.). Follow your physician's instructions; however, continue the lifestyle that supports a natural approach to your womb wellness. The bonus of womb detox is reduction or even elimination of vaginal odor, blood clotting and PMS. All this is an indication that nature is winning on behalf of your womb and that the tumor is losing the war to destroy your womb. Your overall wellness will be improving. You will smile soon. In fact, you will laugh out loud and sing and dance yourself into wellness.

The Making of a Fibroid Tumor

WE ARE WHAT WE EAT, THINK, & FEEL

A tumor is mucus that has formed and accumulated over time through steady consumption of animal proteins, calcium (from dairy) and "Fast Foods."

What Creates A Tumor?

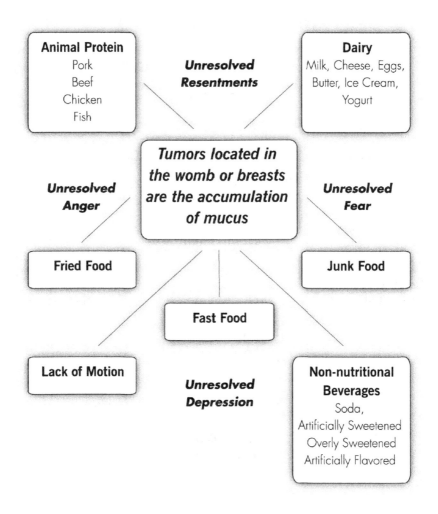

Animal Protein
Pork
Beef
Chicken
Fish

Unresolved Resentments

Dairy
Milk, Cheese, Eggs,
Butter, Ice Cream,
Yogurt

Unresolved Anger

Tumors located in the womb or breasts are the accumulation of mucus

Unresolved Fear

Fried Food

Junk Food

Fast Food

Lack of Motion

Unresolved Depression

Non-nutritional Beverages
Soda,
Artificially Sweetened
Overly Sweetened
Artificially Flavored

The Un-Making of a Fibroid Tumor

WE ARE WHAT WE EAT, THINK, & FEEL

Tumors don't survive without mucus accumulated from consuming animal proteins, calcium (from dairy) and Fast Foods.

What Prevents A Tumor?

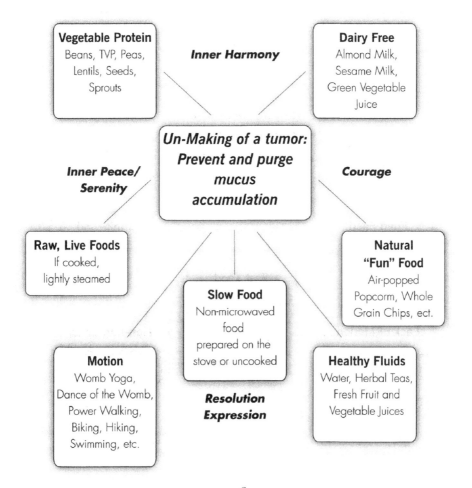

Vegetable Protein
Beans, TVP, Peas, Lentils, Seeds, Sprouts

Inner Harmony

Dairy Free
Almond Milk, Sesame Milk, Green Vegetable Juice

Un-Making of a tumor: Prevent and purge mucus accumulation

Inner Peace/ Serenity

Courage

Raw, Live Foods
If cooked, lightly steamed

Natural "Fun" Food
Air-popped Popcorn, Whole Grain Chips, ect.

Slow Food
Non-microwaved food prepared on the stove or uncooked

Resolution Expression

Motion
Womb Yoga, Dance of the Womb, Power Walking, Biking, Hiking, Swimming, etc.

Healthy Fluids
Water, Herbal Teas, Fresh Fruit and Vegetable Juices

Overcoming a Toxic Lifestyle

If you have this book in your hands, you probably are interested in finding ways to take better care of yourself. Not everyone will decide to become a vegetarian or vegan. However, consider eliminating toxic foods and toxic practices from your life; while raising the frequency of your womb centers. The strategies here focus on Nutrition, Physical Care and Emotional/Mental Care. Perform them daily or weekly as needed for the restoration of wellness to your reproductive womb, the womb of your heart and the womb of your mind.

Nutrition
- **Do** choose the food plan that supports your womb wellness.
- **Do** prepare/eat a meal with a family member/members at least once a week.
- **Do** drink 1 quart of pure water, daily.
- **Do** drink Woman's Life Herbal formula before 12 noon, daily.
- **Do** take in "green" 2- 3X a day. Choose from - organic green vegetable juice, herbal tea, salads and soups.
- **Do** eat vegetable proteins, i.e., beans, peas, lentils, raw nuts (in moderation), seeds and sprouts. Soak seeds, nuts and beans in water overnight.
- **Do** take for calcium: almond, sesame and sunflower milk.
- **Do** take your Green Life Formula which helps to reduce the desire to overeat.
- **Do** consume live foods and beverages in 75% of your diet.

Especially while on a detoxing plan:
- **Don't** eat fried foods and fast foods.
- **Don't** eat meat (if flesh food is consumed – baked fish only in small amounts).
- **Don't** eat processed foods (canned or frozen).
- **Don't** eat white rice, white bread, white pasta, white sugar (or brown sugar).
- **Don't** drink alcoholic or artificially sweetened beverages.

Physical Care
- **Do** head to toe exercise daily: power-walk, stretch, bike, dance, etc.
- **Do** raise your legs against the wall at a 45° for 5-10 minutes in the morning and evening to stimulate circulation and support alignment.
- **Do** take sunrise hot and cold showers and sunset hot baths.
- **Do** take enemas or herbal laxatives or Colon Ease to help release waste from the colon, which causes pain and pressure to the womb.
- **Do** apply a clay pack over your womb center overnight from 3–7 times a week.
- **Do** get a good night's sleep each night to restore your body.
- **Don't** take non-prescription, "entertainment" drugs.
- **Don't** smoke "entertainment" drugs nor tobacco.

Emotional/Mental Care
- **Do** read womb wellness material to reinforce these concepts for your womb life.
- **Do** use oils and gemstones that address your various womb issues, concerns, and goals.
- **Do** refer to texts for dietary support: *Heal Thyself for Health and Longevity; Sacred Woman: The Guide to Healing the Feminine Body, Mind and Spirit* (womb wellness menus and recipes); *and The City of Wellness: Restoring Your Health Through the Seven Kitchens of Consciousness* (liquid and solid meal plans).
- **Do** engage in activities that promote your creativity and wellness.
- **Do** pray and meditate to rejuvenate and raise your frequency of wellness.
- **Do** form "Womb Circles" for sharing and support.
- **Don't** watch non-educational TV.
- **Don't** curse or yell –instead channel hostility into positive creative acts.

GET READY

Get ready to detox and purify for your womb wellness. Prepare yourself and the space around you.

As stated at the opening of this book, if you are presently consulting a physician for existing health challenges, CONTINUE to follow the advice of your physician. The information provided here is designed to be inspirational and help you make informed decisions about your health.

This material is NOT intended to be a substitute for any medical advice or treatment that has been prescribed by your physician.

In the days before you begin a detox plan, prepare you body, mind, spirit and environment for your exciting journey to wellness. Some things to do:

Purchase the wholistic foods and herbs you will need.

Prepare your Kitchen Laboratory.

You will need:
- A juicer to juice live fruits and vegetables
- A blender to blend juices and nutrients
- A stainless steel pot for preparing herbal teas

Prepare your Hydrotherapy Room (bathroom).

You will need:
- A footstool to raise your feet and knees to facilitate elimination
- An enema bag to assist colon cleansing while detoxing

Prepare for your physical fitness.

You will need:
- Sneakers and loose-fitting clothing

Prepare your mind.

- Read material on wellness.

- Your decision to detox should be a private and individual one. As you are detoxing, form Wellness Circles with others who are detoxing for support and fun!

Prepare your spirit.

- Consider prayers and affirmations to recite that are appropriate for you and your wellness goals.

- This is also a good time to meditate about Global Womb Wellness.

Prepare to record your journey to wellness.

- Purchase or prepare a notebook to record your experiences of transformation to wellness of body, mind and spirit.

DAILY WOMB WORK

1. **Align** yourself to wellness. Listen to the Womb Wellness CDs for re-enforcement.

2. **Drink** herbal formulas for 7 to 21 days.
   (Amounts will vary for individuals.)

3. **Avoid fried foods.** They can contribute to heart attacks, high blood pressure and strokes. Instead, eat vegetables steamed 3 to 5 minutes. Nearly one in three US adults has high blood pressure. Since there are no symptoms, nearly one-third have had undiagnosed high blood pressure for years. Untreated and uncontrolled high blood pressure can lead to stroke, heart attack, heart failure, kidney failure. (www.americanheart.org)

4. **Replace dairy products** which contribute to respiratory ills (asthma, hay fever and bronchitis). Instead, obtain proteins and calcium from seed or nut milk and green vegetable juices. Today, more than 35 million Americans are living with diseases such as asthma, emphysema and bronchitis. (www.lungusa.org)

5. **Avoid Sugar** (brown or white) which contributes to arthritis, tooth decay, stress, depression, mood swings and acne. Instead, enjoy soaked dried fruits (currants, raisins, dates, apricots). Processed sugar is deadly. It suppresses the immune system's ability to manufacture antibodies. Sugar depletes B vitamins needed to detoxify the liver, the most important organ in the body-healing process. (www.stopcancer.com)

6. **Drink 8 glasses of room temperature or warm water daily** to prevent dehydration, premature aging and constipation. Dehydration is loss of water and the blood salts: potassium and sodium. Extreme dehydration damages the kidneys, brain and heart.

7. **Drink Green.** A pint of green juice each day helps prevent sluggishness, poor circulation, obesity, cellulite and brittle bones. According to the 1999–2000 National Health & Nutrition Examination Survey (NHANES), more than 64% of US adults are either overweight or obese. Drinking Green Life Formula helps to reduce the desire to overeat, increases your energy, and nourishes your womb.

8. **Reduce animal flesh consumption per week** to half of your present intake. Replace extremely difficult-to-digest animal flesh proteins (pork, beef, lamb, etc.) with skinless organic chicken and fish (not shell fish). Better still is to eat vegetable proteins (beans, peas, lentils, sprouts). For optimal digestion, eat proteins only at midday. If you make these changes, you help minimize and/or prevent cancer, hypertension, constipation and poor circulation. Digesting meat depletes enzymes that are critical to the immune system for fighting cancer cells. Vegetable proteins don't use up those enzymes.

9. **Eat vegetables and fruits daily.** Two servings of salad, soup, broth or steamed vegetables support colon and womb wellness and rejuvenation. One to two servings of fresh fruit promote internal body purity and prevent mucus build-up that can cause sinus congestion, hay fever, colds and tumors.

10. **Take one step at a time.** Consider using the strategies in this section and in **Overcoming a Toxic Lifestyle** in this portal. Remember that it took you some time to develop the conditions that prevent your optimal wellness. It may take some time to change toxic habits and undo womb damage. Be patient with yourself. Love yourself. Trust yourself to choose the strategies and tools that will help you to reclaim balance and wellness. You are on your way; one step at a time.

STEP BY STEP

What step am I on? What steps do I take?

These are basic steps or levels of food consumption. Most people's food plan exists on more than one of them. To detox and rejuvenate try to prepare, eat and drink one step higher than your present level for 1 to 7 days. For optimal wellness follow the **Advanced Juice Fast** for 7 consecutive days, once each season (84 days).

1. **Pre-Beginner and Beginner (Flexitarian):** Right now if you eat meats, cooked foods and other foods that do not entirely support your wellness, your transition from these choices can lead to an increased level of wellness. Begin by eating easier to digest organic chicken and fish (not shell fish). Eventually omit flesh foods (beef, pork, lamb, goat, turkey, chicken, fish). Incorporate whole grains, sprouts, beans, peas, and lentils (soaked in water overnight)into your diet. Consume vegetable protein. Eat greater amounts of fresh fruits and vegetables. Use Natural and Whole Foods to prepare favorite family recipes.

2. **Intermediate (Vegetarian):** Consume only vegetarian foods. Omit all flesh foods (seafood, beef, pork, lamb, turkey, goat, etc.). Fresh vegetable intake should include 50% –75% live raw food and 25-50% cooked food. When cooking vegetables, steam lightly to retain maximum live enzymes and oxygen.

3. **Advanced Intermediate (Vegan):** Consume 100% live, uncooked food. Live foods include organic live proteins (sprouted beans, raw soaked nuts and seeds, avocadoes), salads, live soups, uncooked grains such as couscous, tabouli, bulgur wheat. Consume whole or juiced fresh fruits and vegetables. Drink daily: warm water (8oz. glasses), 5 cups Master Herbal tea and 8oz of Kidney-Liver Flush.

4. **Advanced Juice Fast:** Consume 100% organic liquid meals only. This is usually done for specific periods of time as a cleansing regime. An advanced cleaning regime consists of two vegetable juice meals for rejuvenation and one fruit juice meal for detoxification daily. Additionally, there should be a daily intake of 1/2 gallon warm water (8oz. glasses), 5 cups Master Herbal tea and 8 ozs. of Kidney-Liver flush every day.

NUTRITIONAL PLAN FOR WOMB WELLNESS

The Nutritional Plan below is a suggested guide based on a vegetarian/vegan lifestyle. Think of it as a "starter kit." You are in charge of your wellness. Add or subtract appropriate choices in each category. Plan menus for the week. Shop in advance for ingredients you will need. Whenever possible purchase organic food. Use fresh vegetables and fruits for juicing.

Pre-breakfast
Juice of lemon or lime with warm water

Breakfast
Liquid Breakfast:
8-16 oz. Fresh fruit juice; squeezed(citrus) or juiced

(Wait 30- 60 minutes between eating and drinking)

Solid Breakfast:
Fresh Fruits: whole, chopped, diced, pureed
Whole-grain cereal (optional, with soymilk or nut milk)

Lunch
(Heaviest meal at midday)
Liquid Lunch:
8-16 oz. Fresh vegetable juice

(Wait 30 minutes between eating and drinking)

Solid Lunch:
Protein:
Meat eaters: baked, non-shellfish or chicken (small amount)
Non-meat eaters: beans, peas, lentils, nuts, seeds, sprouts
(Grains, nuts and seeds must be soaked overnight.)

Starch: (Some starches repeated from proteins)
Whole grains, brown rice, corn on the cob, baked potato, tabouli, couscous, millet, wheat or sprouted bread (toasted)

Vegetables:
Raw vegetable salad, blended "live" vegetable soup
Raw or steamed vegetables
(If steaming vegetables, for 3 to 4 minutes only.)
Eat okra three times a week

Dinner
(Lighter than lunch)
Liquid Dinner:
Same as lunch choices

(Wait 30 minutes between eating and drinking)

Solid Dinner:
Protein or starch:
Same as lunch choices
Eat protein or starch at dinner with either steamed or raw
vegetables.

Vegetables:
Same as lunch choices

**Vegetables and herbs to consume raw or steamed or and
juiced:** kale, parsley, turnips, cucumber, scallions, spinach, red
radish, watercress, celery, broccoli

Vegetables and herbs to consume in moderation:
carrots and beets (for those with diabetes)
ginger (for those with high blood pressure)

COLON CONNECTION

The condition of the colon is directly linked to the condition of the womb. For every meal you consume, the body should digest food, assimilate nutrients and eliminate waste. If you consume 3 meals per day, at the end of 7 days you will have consumed 21 meals. You should have 21 bowel movements within the 7 days. If you have only one bowel movement per day for the 21 meals, then the waste of 14 meals is backed up in your colon. This is chronic constipation.

In the state of chronic constipation you might be carrying 5 to 20 lbs. of waste in your colon, which can cause your colon to become prolapsed. When a prolapsed colon presses down on the bladder, it can cause frequent, uncontrollable urination. In time, the weight of the waste compromises wellness in both the colon and bladder. They in turn press on the uterus, causing it to become weak and potentially sexually malfunctioning. Additionally, there may be heavy menstrual bleeding, clotting and cramping.

Perform colon wellness techniques to prevent damages to the womb and the rest of the body. During advanced cleansing, take 1-3 enemas weekly in your hydrotherapy room (bathroom) over a 28-day period.

Colon wellness techniques (also supports womb wellness):
- Drink Kidney-Liver Flush* before breakfast.
- Continue to take enemas periodically.
- While bathing, massage your colon, bladder and womb areas in a clockwise motion.
- If suffering from constipation and/or womb issues, see your colon therapist for professional support.

Directions for taking an enema:
1. Use a 1-2 quart enema bag which resembles a hot water bottle and can be purchased at any pharmacy or drugstore. (Directions will be included in enema kit package.)
2. Fill bag with warm water and an enema implant (listed below) of your choice.
3. Lubricate the tip of the insert nozzle with a personal lubricating jelly.
4. While either sitting or standing, gently insert nozzle into rectum and release clamp on the hose.

5. Allow the water to slowly enter your colon. When you feel full, fasten the clamp on the hose to stop the flow of water. Massage the abdomen to further provoke waste to loosen.

6. Then release the clamp and allow the water to flow again.

7. When ready to release, remove the nozzle from the rectum. Sit on the toilet.

8. For greater elimination, sit in a squatted position or put one foot or both feet on a stool placed in front of the toilet.

9. Repeat steps 3 to 8 until the enema bag is empty.

10. As you progress with your cleansing, you will be able to retain a quart of water for a longer period of time before elimination.

Add any one of these implants to the water in the enema bag:

- 1oz. wheatgrass (rejuvenation)

- 3 Tbsp. liquid chlorophyll (rejuvenation)

- Juice of lemon or lime (releases mucus, gas)

- 3 Tbsp. organic apple cider vinegar (same benefit as lemon/lime)

- 1/4 tsp. of strained goldenseal (cleansing)

For Kidney-Liver Flush recipe see Herbs.

DARE TO DETOX!

*D*etoxification is the process of getting rid of toxins. It took some time to develop tumors and other symptoms of dis-ease. It will take time to undo the damage.

*B*e prepared. For at least a week before you begin a fasting regimen, eat a light vegetarian diet. This will make it easier to begin the actual fast. Plan ahead for meals and responsibilities to minimize interruptions to your detox efforts.

*B*e consistent. Once you begin your fast, consume only vegetable and fruit juices and live food; follow the exercise, breathing, and resting instructions for your fast. Very soon your body (and your womb) will start getting rid of accumulated toxins. Be patient.

*D*on't be alarmed. As your body begins to detox, you may experience one or more fasting crises. This means your body is having a reaction to the cleansing process. These reactions are natural. Your body is getting rid of the toxins; you are detoxing. You can minimize or prevent fasting crises or detox drama, if you prepare as suggested above. Don't panic. Don't stop cleansing. Below are some of the ways your body may react in the first few days of your fast:

Fasting Crises

headaches	dizziness	heavy breathing
tiredness	flatulence	skin eruptions
mental confusion	blood pressure rising	aches & pains
vaginal discharges	physical weakness	blurred vision
fevers, chills	nightmares	shortness of breath
impatience	sadness, crying	mood swings

These and similar reactions come from a history of eating too much starch, sugar, heavy meats, fried foods and dairy products, regularly. The detoxing reactions you may experience can last from an hour or two to a couple of days.
Don't panic.
Don't stop detoxing.

Be patient. To help your body adjust to detoxification crises:

1. Discontinue drinking fruit juices until the symptoms subside. Drink only vegetable juice combinations to stabilize and strengthen the body before re-introducing fruit juices.

2. Immediately take an enema, using only warm water in a quart-sized enema bag.

3. Discontinue taking salt baths for two days and take warm showers instead.

4. Give yourself a vigorous massage, starting at your feet and working upwards toward your heart; or have a professional massage.

5. Discontinue taking Kidney-Liver Flush and replace it with the juice of one lemon, three tsp. of cold-pressed olive oil and eight ounces of warm water. Also drink a mixture of dandelion and alfalfa tea (2 tsp. of each herb to 2 cups of water).

6. Get more rest and sleep.

Follow these instructions, and the uncomfortable reactions to cleansing should be over within one to three days. If the symptoms persist, contact your fasting consultant. Remember, you are engaged in a Womb Revolution. Revolution is change. Expect resistance.

Be courageous. Prepare to wage a successful campaign to restore wellness to your womb and your life. Examine the tools and strategies on the following pages.

Relax. You have choices.

Choices

*I*n order to wage a successful campaign to restore wellness to your womb and your life, you will need to follow a nutritional plan for detoxification and reju- venation. (See: Nutritional Plan for Womb Wellness) and attend to the well- ness of your colon. (See: The Colon Connection). You will also need tools and strategies.

The following are time-tested and well-womb proven tools and strategies for detoxing and rejuvenating your reproductive womb, the womb of your heart and the womb of your mind. Think of them as a banquet of suggestions to support you in your quest for wellness.

Don't try to do and use everything on the first day or even on the last day of your 28-day detox schedule. It is one thing to challenge yourself to do your best. However, it is completely another thing to do stress-causing things (even in the name of wellness).

Make choices: You don't have to do everything in each category. Find what res- onates with your lifestyle and your wellness goals. You may decide not to explore a particular therapy at this time. That's fine.

Pay attention to your reactions and needs. If you have diabetes or high blood pressure, use apple cider vinegar instead of Epsom salts in your bath. If you need to rest after taking an enema, take it before going to bed, not before going to work.

Make adjustments. A cup of herb tea might not be your cup of tea. Instead mix your herbs into your salad. If you sprinkle herbs into your bath, your skin—your largest organ—will drink them right in!

Add strategies that support your new wellness lifestyle. You have choices: ele- ments, baths, affirmations, herbs and more.

Empower yourself to gloriously overcome an angry vagina.

Take care of yourself. Do, YOU!

TOOLS AND STRATEGIES

Tools

Elements: Combine the elements: Ether, Air, Fire, Water and Earth with baths, massages, tonics and packs to promote balance and support your wellness.

Clay: Queen Afua Rejuvenation Green Clay Formula V. Clay is a body food made up of calcium, magnesium, potassium and zinc. Green Clay can be used internally and externally to soothe swollen/painful areas of the body – apply as needed.

Herbs (Plants and Bulbs): In ancient cultures, most cures and remedies were made from plants. Herbs, plants and bulbs are proven wellness tools.

Gemstones: Records from the earliest history of humanity show that gemstones have long been used as tools to promote spiritual, emotional and physical wellness.

Essential oils: Like herbs, essential oils from plants have been used for thousands of years as restoratives to the wellness of body, mind, and spirit.

Implants, Packs and Poultices: "Tools" you create, usually by making a paste of containing herbs and/or green clay and/or organic olive oil or castor oil. The paste is then wrapped in a piece of gauze or cheesecloth and placed on or into a specific area for the purpose of drawing out toxins and aiding wellness restoration.

Soaks and washes: Use herbs and/or green clay to create a liquid solution to include in the bath or for washing or soaking a specific area of the body.

Wellness-promoting beverages: Drinks, teas, formulas and tonics.

Water: To flush impurities, drink at least eight glasses of room temperature-to-warm water daily. For drinking and making wellness beverages, use the purest form of water available to you.

Strategies

Hydrotherapy:
- **Baths, Showers, Sweat and Steam sessions:** for relaxing and relieving stress and removing toxins that have been purged to the skin surface; taken 3 – 7x weekly.
- **Enemas:** to remove toxins from colon – done personally, 2 – 3X weekly.
- **Colonics:** to more thoroughly remove waste from your colon – done by colonic therapist, 2 – 8x per season (84 days) based on individual's wellness level.

Physical Work:
- **Exercise:** Individual choice, such as stretching, walking, yoga, or dancing at least 30 minutes daily for full body benefits. (Be sure to see POR-TAL FIVE – CELEBRATION for Dance of the Womb and Womb Yoga.)
- **Body Massages:** Massage the pressure points of your face, hands and feet as you shower and bathe and apply body lotions. Massage pressure points throughout the day especially to relieve stress. Arrange to receive a professional massage at least once a month. Also, consider exchanging massages with a family member or close friend.
- **Womb Massages:** Daily, massage womb center in a clockwise motion.

Mind and Heart Work:
- **Meditations and Affirmations:** Strategies for restoring the womb of the mind (thoughts) and the womb of the heart (emotions) go hand in hand with caring for physical body.

Communicate with yourself:
- **Journaling:** Take time to write down in a notebook or diary your positive and negative experiences, especially during an extended detox regimen. (7–28 day fast or full-season cleansing program).

Communicate with others:
- **Womb Circles and Gatherings:** Sharing Share experiences with others also on the path of overcoming an angry vagina, a toxic lifestyle.

ELEMENTS

$\mathcal{T}$he body is made of elements that are present on the earth. As a result, we can use these natural elements in nature to heal ourselves. The relationship of the elements to the body and spirit are:

Ether — Mind

Air — Lungs

Fire: — Blood; Reproductive organs

Water — 75% of the body consists of this element alone

Earth — Bones and teeth; colon

The following purification exercises are designed to enlist the benefits of the natural elements.

*Ether * Air * Fire * Water * Earth assist to promote balance and support your wellness.

Proper use of the elements will help you be in harmony with nature, the universe, and all your relations.

Each exercise incorporates several tools and strategies. I suggest that, as you become familiar with them, you try to adopt and adapt the activities that support your wellness.

*Note:
If you have high blood pressure, avoid salt baths, ginger and tea, and cranberry juice. Use apple cider vinegar instead of bath salts. If diabetes or high blood pressure challenges presently prevent you from using an ingredient suggested in these exercises, prepare a vegetable green drink and/or consult the herbs section for appropriate substitutes. Follow precautions prescribed by your physician.

Womb Wellness Liberation Exercise (Ether Element)

1. Sit in a chair.
2. Center yourself in Wellness. Allow your mind and your body to become one.
3. Breathe deeply. Allow your breath to become one with your womb center.
4. Move to a comfortable flat surface (your bed or the floor).
5. Place both legs against the wall in a 45° angle. If you have high blood

pressure, place legs on 3 pillows for a more gentle inversion. Keep legs elevated for 10–15 minutes.

6. Massage your forehead in circular motions 9 times as you inhale and exhale, slowly.

7. Massage your heart area in circular motions 9 times as you inhale and exhale, slowly.

8. Massage your womb center in circular motions 9 times as you inhale and exhale, slowly.

9. Clear your mind. Let go of womb trauma, drama, and suffering that is part of your negative past.

10. While massaging your womb centers, recite affirmations.

Affirmations:

I am massaging away past pain and resentment. (Breathe deeply.)
I accept peace, power, and joy into my life! (Breathe fully.)

Womb Wellness Bath (Water/ Ether/Fire Elements)

1. Run a hot bath, and place one or more of the following wellness tools into the tub of water:

   • 1 hand-sized rose quartz stone –for a self-love charge
   • 1 hand-sized clear quartz stone –for clarity and purification
   • 3 – 4 drops of cleansing sage and lotus oil –for "sweating" your spirit
   • 2 Tbsp. of Dead Sea Salt(See *Note above) –for cleansing your auric (energy) field
   • 1 cup of freshly pressed ginger (See *Note above) – for circulation
   • A handful of hyssop herbs for detoxing the spirit
   • 2 – 3 handfuls of pink or white rose petals for beautifying the Womb of your Heart

2. Turn off bright lights and replace with a soft, low light or candlelight

3. Before entering the tub and/or while bathing recite affirmations.

4. Repeat affirmations several times as you release and replenish yourself. This bath will soothe you and aid in the release of overall physical and spiritual trauma.

5. Luxuriate in tub for 30 to 60 minutes.

   Affirmations:
   I am detoxing my life of hurt, fear, and resentment.
   (Breathe deeply.)

   > *I am taking a bath to reconnect to my natural beauty.*
   > *(Breathe fully.)*

Womb Wellness Shower (Water/Ether Elements)

1. Take a shower and let the water run over your entire body which houses your womb centers: the womb of the mind, the womb of the heart, and the womb of your Sacred Seat (vagina).
2. Before entering the shower and while showering recite affirmations.
   Affirmation:
   I release all angry vagina symptoms from my body, mind, and spirit. (Breathe fully.)
   I am taking this shower to nurture myself into tranquility. (Breathe deeply.)

Womb Wellness Air Bath (Air/Ether Elements)

1. After bathing, lovingly dry your body.
2. Sit or lie down in a quiet, restful place. Take a 10–15 minute air bath. Allow the air to caress your womb centers.
3. Wrap yourself in a non-constricting, free-flowing garment made of natural organic fabric.
4. While air-bathing, recite affirmations.
   Affirmations:
   I am taking an air bath to reconnect to my natural beauty. (Breathe fully.)
   I am soothing my spirit and removing hurt, fear, and resentment from my life. (Breathe fully.)

Womb Wellness Herbal Tonic (Water/Ether Elements)

1. Prepare an herbal tea or green drink. Chose an herb or vegetables for your green drink that supports the detoxification and rejuvenation of a womb issue you want to address.

2. While bathing or in a quite restful environment drink your tea or green juice from a bowl or gourd. The bowl represents wholeness of body, mind, and spirit.

   Affirmations:

   I am drinking these herbs to detox hurt, fear, and resentment from my life. (Breathe deeply.)

   I drink wholeness, peace, calm, and vitality into my womb center. (Breathe internally.)

Womb Wellness Fire Tonic and Fire Pack (Fire/Ether Elements)

1. Prepare a hot castor oil pack and pour 8 – 16 ozs. ginger tea or unsweetened cranberry juice. (See *Note above)

2. Drink the ginger tea or unsweetened cranberry juice.

3. Lie down in a quiet, restful place and place the hot castor oil pack over the womb area. Place a heating pad over the hot oil pack on your womb for 30 to 60 minutes.

4. While the heating pad and hot oil pack are on your womb area, recite your affirmations.

   Affirmations:

   Fire elements support me as I burn away all womb sorrows. (Breathe fully.)

   I am igniting my own wellness and joy. (Breathe deeply.)

Womb Wellness Earth Pack (Earth /Ether Elements)

1. Prepare an Outer Womb Pack and an Inner Womb Pack.

   Outer Womb Pack: Spread a 1 Tbsp. of clay 1 inch thick into a square of gauze or cheese-cloth about the size of your two hands. Fold gauze into a package to place over your womb area.

   Inner Womb Pack: Put 1/4 spoon of clay on a small square of gauze. Roll the clay and gauze into a small tube-shaped insert to be placed inside your vagina.

2. For advanced cleansing, prepare and drink 8 ozs. of Clay Tonic (1 Tbsp. of green clay blended with 8 ozs. of water)

3. Urinate before applying clay treatments.

4. Lie down on your bed. Insert the Inner Clay Pack into your vagina a few inches deep. Place the Outer Clay Pack on your womb area. Overnight the clay packs will draw out impurities and rejuvenate the womb.

5. While applying the clay packs recite your affirmations.

6. In the morning take a hot water shower and remove both packs.

   Affirmations:

   Earth elements support me as I draw out all womb impurities. (Breathe internally.)

   I am rejuvenating my womb to wholeness, health, and happiness. (Breathe fully.)

Womb-Soul Sweat (Ether/Air/ Fire/Water/Earth Elements)

Weekly or biweekly, perform a Womb-Soul Sweat at your local bathhouse or spa that has sauna and/or steam rooms. The Womb-Soul Sweat incorporates the use of all five elements.

At the bathhouse:

1. Shower your entire body.
2. Sweat for 10–15 minutes in wet steam room or dry heat sauna.
3. While sweating, self-massage your thighs and pelvic area with olive oil and castor oil.
4. Rest for 5 minutes outside the heat room. While resting, allow the air to caress your womb centers. (Remain wrapped in a robe or cloth so you do not get a chill.)
5. Repeat 10–15 minutes in sauna or steam rooms.
6. Take hot and cold showers between sweats.
7. Throughout sweat/rest rotations, drink water with fresh-squeezed lemon juice or herbal tea or organic green juice.
8. Repeat 1–6 sweats for 1–2 hours
9. Follow your bathhouse visit by applying Inner and Outer Clay Packs overnight. Take a hot shower in the morning.
10. While sweating, showering and resting recite affirmations.

    Affirmations:

    I offer love and forgiveness for all my relationships; they are born out of me. (Breathe fully.)

    Today, I release anger from my womb. My destiny is liberation! I am free! (Breathe deeply.)

HERBS

(Plants and Bulbs)

*I*n ancient cultures most cures and remedies were made from plants. Even up to the present millennium, around the globe women's medicine chests contain vials of tinctures from flowers, jars of salves from plants and bundles of dried roots, stems and leaves to be turned into herbal beverages, soaks and washes.

(Gerianne's "Godmother Betty" (now, an ancestor), was an avid fan of chickweed herb. She would make a chickweed solution and apply it to the infected area for quick relief and elimination of skin irritations. She highly praised chickweed washes for everything from diaper rashes to vaginal douching.)

The following herbal and natural remedies can be used to support the womb wellness and related issues, particularly during your 28-Day Womb Detox Fast. Use 2 or 3 of these herbs daily according to your needs. Beyond your fast continue to include appropriate herbs as tools to support your wellness strategies.

Preparation of Herbs

- **Loose herbs:** Use 1 tsp. of herbs to 1 cup of water. Boil water, then turn off flame and add loose herbs to pot.

- **Powered herbs:** Use 1/4 tsp. of powered herbs to 1 cup of hot water.

- **Herbal tinctures and nonalcoholic herbal extracts:** Use 10 drops to 1 cup of water.

All the herbs I have recommended are grown on Mother Earth.

Allow herbs to steep from 2 hours to overnight. Prepare 3 cups for average daily use.

Use and drink organically-grown herbs, not sweetened juice-drinks with herbal names.

ALOE VERA

(For general wellness; mild bowel regulator; soothing, moisturizing)

- Make a tonic for general wellness by blending 1–2 Tbsp. aloe pulp/ juice/gel with fruit or vegetable juice to make a tonic. Drink 2 -3x a day. Taking *Aloe Vera internally* has been linked to the improved blood glucose levels in diabetics.

- Make a poultice for scraps or cuts. Make a wash for minor burns and skin irritations. Clean area appropriately. You can also use the actual plant leaf split open or aloe gel or liquid to apply topically to affected area to soothe and moisturize.

Affirmation:
I am using this aloe to soothe my hurts and promote my wellness.

CAYENNE

(Stimulates blood circulation)

- Cayenne, one of the ingredients in Kidney-Liver Flush, stimulates blood circulation in the womb and the entire body.

- Add a pinch of cayenne to vegetable juice.

Affirmation:
I stimulate the blood in my womb and accept only what brings joy and positive fulfillment to my life.

CHICKWEED

(Relieves skin irritations)

- Drink chickweed as a tea for internal cleansing and general wellbeing,

- Use chickweed in implant, poultice or pack form for relieving vaginal itching.

- Use a chickweed to make a as a wash or a soak solution for use I the vaginal area.

Affirmation:
I am whole I will allow no one to be an irritation to my soul.

COMFREY

(Relieves inflammation, especially swollen breasts)

- Make a poultice combining steeped comfrey leaves and green clay in cheesecloth. Apply over swollen breasts over night to relieve inflammation.

- For vaginal discharge make a comfrey solution by boiling 1 quart of water and steep 4 Tbsp. of comfrey herbs in the water overnight. Wash the vagina with a clean cloth that has been soaked in the comfrey solution.

Affirmation:
As I renew myself, my breasts and my womb I am nourished in nature by the light and the love of the Creator.

DANDELION

(For strengthening the blood, especially anemia produced from excessive menstrual flow)

- Steep and drink dandelion tea to help strengthen the blood. (Similar results from drinking Alfalfa tea or Sorrel.)

- Related suggestions: Eat green vegetables and drink green juices. Add 1–2 Tbsp. of wheat grass or spirulina to green juice. Stop poisoning your blood with processed, toxic junk food and fast food.

Affirmation:
I cast out all toxins no matter how large or small. I trust the Creator to make me whole.

ECHINACEA

(For use when cancerous womb is present)

- Steep and drink Echinacea tea. Take for up to 16 weeks -4 menstrual cycles).

- Related suggestions for this and most female *dis*-eases: Drink 8–12 oz. of **unsweetened** cranberry juice daily. Drink 1 pint of green vegetable juice daily. Fast. Take herbal enemas and laxatives.

Affirmation:
This herb is a gift. I use it today, for restoration and rejuvenation.

FENUGREEK

(For use when inflamed uterus is present)

- Steep and drink Fenugreek tea. Take for up to 16 weeks - 4 menstrual cycles).

- Related suggestions: Use clay packs 7 days. Take wheat grass douche 1–2 oz. for 3 to 7 days.

- Eat and drink live foods and juices.

Affirmation:
This herb is a gift. I will allow no one and nothing to inflame me, nor prevent my wellness.

GARLIC BULB

(Nature's helper for fighting infections)

- Place a clove of garlic in cheese cloth and use as a vaginal implant (suppository). Leave implanted for 2 hours.

- Related suggestions: Use clay packs for 7 days. Take wheat grass douche 1– 2 oz. for 3 to 7 days. Use Lemon or Lime douche with 1/4 teaspoon of aloe powder. Eat a flesh-free diet (vegetarian and fruit) for an alkaline womb.

Affirmation:
I will not gossip! I will keep sweet thoughts and speak loving words so that my words will reflect in kind the sacredness of my womb center.

GINGER

(For blood circulation; relieves nausea)

- Boil 3–4 cups of water; turn off flame. Steep 1 tsp. of grated ginger root or 1/2 tsp. of powdered ginger per cup. Drink ginger tea as a refreshing aid for stimulating blood circulation and warming the body – especially, the hands and feet. Ginger tea is known for properties when taken to relieve cold and flu symptoms. Ginger tea also curbs nausea (as related to morning sickness and motion sickness) and helps to eliminate gas.

- **Do not take ginger** if you are using blood thinners or have a bleeding disorder or have gallbladder disease.

Affirmation:
It is time to active womb wellness. I drink this herb to warm myself and to active my womb wellness.

MARSHMALLOW

(For vaginal burning)

- Steep herb and use tea to prepare a vaginal douche.

- Related suggestions: Use clay packs for 7 days. Drink Green Juice Daily.

Affirmation:
I release my anger as I use this herb to cleanse. I am cleansing my life.

OAT STRAW

(For menstrual cramps)

- Make a clay poultice. Place poultice over pelvis for 2 hours. Steep and drink a cup of Oat Straw tea.

- Related suggestions: Avoid eating starch and protein a week before menses and during your menstrual flow. Consume fruits and vegetables and herbal teas and water.

Affirmation:
I embrace this womb cycle journey. I release the tensions that create stressful cramps, clots and discomfort during my period.

RED CLOVER

(For womb tone rejuvenation)

- Take a Red Clover sitz bath* 3–4 times a week to tone muscles of pelvic womb area. Steep and drink a cup of Red clover tea daily.

- Related suggestions: massage your womb area, daily in circular pattern. Use clay packs with gauze over pelvic overnight 3–7 times per week for 28 days. Take hot and cold pelvic showers daily.

Affirmation:
I deserve to be toned, fit and rejuvenated.

RED RASPBERRY

(For relaxing the womb)

- Steep and drink Red Raspberry tea to relax the uterine area and in order to enhance fertility.

- Related suggestions: Drink 1–2 Tbsp. of wheat grass or spirulina three times a day with green vegetable juice. Unclog the womb with a Natural Living Lifestyle. Have regular massage work done. Perform Dance of the Womb Movement and/or Womb Yoga at least 30 to 60 minutes a day.

Affirmation:
I release all malice out of my ovaries so that they may be clean and pure.

ROSEMARY

(For symptoms of menopause)

- Steep and drink Rosemary tea to help prevent and/or eliminate hot flashes caused by hormonal imbalances

- Related suggestions: Take 1–2 Tbsp. of spirulina or wheat grass 3x daily with fresh vegetable juice.

Affirmation:
I celebrate the autumn of my life. It is a time of wisdom, spiritual freedom and profound growth.

SAGE

(For blocked menses and to stop the flow of breast milk)

- Steep and drink Sage tea to help to alleviate pre-menopausal systems; such as depression and anxiety. Clary Sage is a known source of natural estrogen, it helps to regulate cells and balance the hormones.

- Related suggestions: Use clay packs and castor oil packs 3–4 times weekly. Fast 4–7 days monthly. Massage yourself daily, (upward towards the heart) with equal parts of castor oil and pure cold pressed olive oil upward towards the heart.

Affirmation:
I open my life and womb to the glory, goodness and abundance that is my birthright as a child on the Divine.

SHEPHERD'S PURSE

(To relieve heavy bleeding):

- Use 10 drops of Shepherd's Purse extract in 8 oz. of warm water twice a day (morning and evening to relieve heavy bleeding.

- Related suggestions: Reduce consumption of flesh-food. Heavy eating of animal protein can contribute to heavy menstrual bleeding and clotting. Eat plenty of grapefruits and oranges, especially the white fiber of the fruit to help flush the womb. Saturate your diet with green food and green juices.

Affirmation:
I support the gentle and nonviolent cleansing of my womb. I am well.

SLIPPERY ELM

(For relief from vaginal itching and burning)

- Make a vaginal implant (suppository) of green clay and steeped slippery elm leaves. Insert implant into your vagina for 2 hours.

- Related suggestions: Eat green vegetables and drink green juices. Prepare and use a chickweed vaginal douche.

Affirmation:
I am whole I will allow no one to be an irritation to my soul. I release them and let them go.

SWEET MEADOW

(Nature's helper to ease symptoms of endometriosis)

- Prepare tea of Meadowsweet herbs. Drink tea to reduce tissue inflammation, gastritis and intestinal discomfort that hinder womb wellness. Related suggestions: Meadowsweet tea is also suggested for relieving discomfort in the kidneys and bladder

- Related suggestions: Drink 2 Tbsp. of soaked flaxseed with warm lemon water regularly.

- **Note: Meadowsweet should not be used if you have asthma or breathing difficulties.**

Affirmation:
I discharge out of my womb all which is not truth and right. I encourage wellness.

WHITE WILLOW

(Nature's helper to ease discomfort)

- Prepare tea of White Willow bark and drink to relieve symptoms of headaches and conditions associated with inflammation, fever and sore muscles.

- Related suggestions: Take 1–2 Tbsp. of green supplements in the form of wheat grass or spirulina or blue green manna 3 times a day with a pint of green juice. Take 2,400 IU of Vitamin E once a day. Drink 2 Tbsp. of soaked flaxseed with warm lemon water.

Affirmation:
I strive to hear the voice of my womb and enjoy my stillness. I will be patient and allow her time to heal.

WOOD BETONY

(Relaxant; tonic)

- Prepare tea by steeping 1–2 tsp. of the herb in boiling water. Drink a cup for relief of headaches, nervous tension, menstrual discomfort and to cleanse the system. Hot wood betony has been found to be useful to relieve extreme discomfort that may occur during difficult labor and child birth.

- Related suggestions: Prepare a Wood Betony poultice to apply to mouth sores. Gargle with a Wood Betony solution to relieve sore throat and sore gum discomforts.

Affirmation:
I allow my head, heart, and womb to open up and give birth and set myself and my baby free to experience a loving delivery experience.

LEMON VERBENA

(For symptoms of fevers, colds; nausea and digestion discomfort)

- Prepare tea by steeping Lemon Verbena herbs in boiling water. Drink a cup as a coolant for fevers, as well as, for relief of symptoms of nausea and digestion discomfort. Drinking Lemon Verbena can offer soothing and calming relief for one in an agitated or nervous state.

- Related suggestions: Try to incorporate Natural Living Lifestyle. Maintain your colon wellness. Do exercises to strengthen the womb of your body and the womb of your mind.

Affirmation:
I am at peace with the womb of my body, the womb of my heart and the womb of my mind. I approach my wellness with calm joy.

CLAY

*G*reen clay is an organic material that is made up of essential minerals, iron oxides and decomposed plant matter. Also known as illite, this clay was named green clay because it is really and naturally green in color. Green clay has been used for detoxification and rejuvenation for centuries. It can be taken both externally and internally. Its many absorbent properties make it an excellent tool for detoxification strategies. Green Clay is a body food made up of calcium, magnesium, potassium and zinc.

In the Queen Afua Rejuvenation Green Clay Formula V, I have enhanced these naturally-occurring minerals with the infusion of essential oils: Red Clover, Eucalyptus Oil, Peppermint Oil and distilled water. Because of the green clay ingredient in this formula, this product can be useful for womb rejuvenation. There are global testimonies about the use of green clay in relieving heartburn, indigestion, diarrhea, as well as, women-related issues, such as, menstrual cramps and morning sickness.

Below is a chart with 21 ways to use Queen Afua Rejuvenation Green Clay Formula V. As said before, the wellness of the womb can be compromised by the unwellness of another part of the body. This chart is to help you to care for your womb wellness as you care for your other parts.

Affirmation: *I go straight to the Mother –Earth– and she will help me to draw toxicity from my body and nourish my wellness.*

Clay Tools and Strategies

Clay Pack or Poultice
Spread a 1 Tbsp. of clay 1 inch thick into a square of gauze or cheesecloth about the size of your two hands. Fold gauze into a package to place over the desired area.

Clay Implant
Put 1/4 spoon of clay on a small square of gauze. Roll the clay and gauze into a small tube-shaped insert to be placed inside your vagina.

Clay Tonic
For advanced cleansing and rejuvenating: Blend 1–2 Tbsp. of green clay into 8 ozs. of pure water or fresh fruit or vegetable juice. You really can get used to the taste of this minty refreshing tonic. the liver.

CLAY WORKS

Green Clay is a body food made up of calcium, magnesium, potassium and zinc. Clay can be used internally and externally. Clay Application: Generously apply clay over area you are working on. Allow clay to dry thoroughly. To remove clay use warm water in a shower or bath. Or use a washcloth and warm water from the sink to remove clay.

Anatomy	Benefits	Application Time (When appropriate, rinse clay after times suggested for each below.)	How to use
Scalp	Itchy Scalp, Hair Loss	2-3 hrs / overnight	Wash hair with natural, shampoo. Apply and massage clay damp hair into hair, cover with white towel.
Face	Pimples & black-heads, toxic aging lines	30 minutes	Wash face with warm water, dry and apply clay.
Eyes	Red eyes, puffy eyes, tired eyes	2 hours	Apply clay with eye gauze.
Ears	Faint hearing, ear wax build-up.	24 hours	Apply gauze behind of and in front of ear.
Gums	Bleeding gums, gum disease	5–10 minutes	Pack a tablespoon of clay over gums, massage and rinse.
Teeth	Plaque/bacteria build-up,	3 minutes	Brush teeth with clay as a natural toothpaste.
Thyroid	Enlarged thyroid	Overnight	Apply with gauze.
Bones & Joints	Shoulders, elbows, hands, hip bones, knees, ankles, feet	Overnight	Apply with gauze.
Lungs	Asthma, short-ness of breath	Overnight	Apply with gauze over lungs.
Boils	Draws out mucus	Overnight	Apply with gauze over boils.

Anatomy	Benefits	Application Time (When appropriate, rinse clay after times suggested for each below.)	How to use
Breasts	Breast tumors, cysts	2-3 hrs/overnight	Apply with gauze over breast.
Kidneys	Water Retention	4 hours	Apply with gauze over kidneys.
Womb	Pain, fibroid tumors, cysts, Vaginal discharge, itching	Overnight 2 hours	Apply with gauze over womb area. Insert 1 teaspoon of clay with cotton swab or make and use a vaginal insert.
Liver	Assists in cleansing of blood	Overnight	Apply with gauze over the liver.
Bladder	Soothes urinary inflammation	4 hours	Apply with gauze over the bladder.
Feet	Pulls out toxins trapped the body through sweat glands of feet	Overnight	Apply clay to feet and toes. Put on clean white cotton socks.
Internal Use	Pain throughout the body	Blend and drink	Blend 1 tablespoon with 8 oz. of water/juice.
Hands	Rejuvenates, softens	Overnight	Apply clay to hands and fingers. Put on clean white cotton gloves.
Male Genitals	Draws out bacteria	Overnight	Apply to genital. Cover with gauze.
Skin	Radiant skin; removes pimples, blackheads	5 minutes	Massage clay into skin with loofa brush or sponge
Sinus	Clears sinus blockage.	30 minutes	Apply over sinus

Essential Oils

Essential oils (EO), like herbal remedies, have been used globally, for thousands of years to rejuvenate the wellness of body, mind, and spirit. These highly concentrated oils are distilled from flowers, trees, bushes and roots. Essential Oils have properties and benefits to similar their cousins, Herbal Remedies. Again, for best results I highly suggest that you use oils that come from plants that are grown organically.

An essential oil can be an antiseptic, stimulant and/or calmative and simultaneously be delightfully aromatic. As I continue to serve my clients with a wholistic, Natural Living approach to wellness, I am pleased to see that Essential Oils are being rediscovered and respected by a whole new generation of wellness-seekers. This could be a sign that we really are trying to, "Go green"!!

The following Essential Oils are listed for their properties and benefits as associated with the womb centers: the Womb of the Mind (thoughts) the Womb of the Heart (emotions) and the Womb of the Sacred Seat (reproductive Womb). explore how these gifts from Mother Nature's garden you can help you to rejuvenate your Womb Wellness.

Strategies for use with Essential Oils

For personal hygiene and beauty:
- Add a few drops of appropriate EO to shampoo and body lotions.

For the body:
- Add a few drops of appropriate EO to bathwater.

- Add a few drops of appropriate to clay pack or poultice. Place over womb or breasts.

As facial steam:
- Add a few drops of EO to facial steamer or into a bowl with hot water. Use a towel over your head like a tent. Place your face over the steam at a safe distance from the hot water

As a mask for face and other skin areas:
- Blend a few drops of EO with green clay and apply to area. Leave on for 5–15 minutes. Wash off in shower or sink with warm water.

As massage oil:
- Add a few drops of EO to olive oil and use to massage the pelvic area.

As an inhalant:
- Follow directions for facial steam.

- Place a few drops of EO on a handkerchief or piece if fabric you like. Tuck into your purse.

For household use:
- Create small sachet pillows made of herbs and infused with a few drops of Essential Oils.

- Make or purchase larger pillows for use in your home. Infuse them with a few drops of EO.

- Put a few drops of EO in a diffuser to mix with steamand scent the room.

- Put a few drops of EO on air vent in the room

- Add several drops of EO to water in a spray bottle. Spray the room.

- Add a few drops of EO to products for cleaning and refreshing laundry, dishes and house wares.

Be creative!

Enjoy the aromas!

Enjoy yourself and your Womb Wellness!

BERGAMOT

Traditional use: Antiseptic used for skin disorders; Aphrodisiac

- **Related Womb Wellness: Heart Womb – Establishes protection**
- **Application:** Add drops to hair and skin lotions.

Affirmation:
I am protected within my own skin. My heart and all of me deserves to be well.

CINNAMON

Traditional use: Cleansing, deodorizing; helpful with diabetes and lowering cholesterol

- **Related Womb Wellness: Mind Womb, Heart Womb – Encourages clarity of emotions**
- **Application:** Use in aromatic sachets for home or personal use.
- **Note: Avoid Cinnamon Oil if you have high blood pressure.**

Affirmation:
I have sweet, clear thoughts. I attract sweet, clear relationships.

EUCALYPTUS

Traditional use: Cleansing, deodorizing: To relieve asthma, sore throat, coughs

- **Related Womb Wellness: Mind Womb – Encourages clarity of thoughts**
- **Application:** Use in baths and for soaks.

Affirmation:
My thoughts are clear. I am not choked or clogged. I can move forward and be well.

FRANKINCENSE

Traditional use: To relieve inflammatory diseases; in perfume and incense

- **Related Womb Wellness: Mind Womb, Heart Womb – Encourages love and goodness**
- **Application:** Use aromatically in home or for personal perfume

Affirmation:

My life is whole. My life is the fragrant with wellness.

GINGER

Traditional use: To soothe Menstrual cramps; Aphrodisiac

- **Related Womb Wellness: Reproductive Womb, Heart Womb – Unblocks fear of joy**
- **Application:** Use to perfume lotions, shampoos and baths

Affirmation:

My life is whole and not cramped. My life is the fragrant and full with wellness.

LAVENDER

Traditional use: To soothe nervous tension; To cleanse home and body; Aphrodisiac

- **Related Womb Wellness: Mind Womb, Heart Womb – Cleanses to receive joy**
- **Application:** Use to perfume lotions, shampoos and baths. Use incense.

Affirmation:

My life is whole. My life is the fragrant with wellness

LEMON

Traditional use: To cleanse body and home

- **Related Womb Wellness: Mind Womb, Heart Womb – Cleanses for clarity**
- **Application:** Add drops to shampoos and baths. Use in home cleaning solutions.

Affirmation:

My home is clean, my heart and mind are clean. I enjoy achieving my wellness.

ROSE

Traditional use: As a perfume

- **Related Womb Wellness: Heart Womb – Encourages beauty and love**
- **Application:** Add drops to shampoos and baths. Use as personal perfume.

Affirmation:

I radiate the fragrance of love. My heart is open to receiving love and wellness.

ROSEMARY

Traditional use: To soothe muscle soreness

- **Related Womb Wellness: Mind Womb, Heart Womb –Soothes thoughts and emotions**
- **Application:** Add drops to baths and body lotions.
- **Note: Avoid Rosemary Oil when pregnant or breastfeeding.**

Affirmation:

My limbs and thoughts and emotions are free to move. I celebrate my wellness.

SAGE

Traditional use: To relieve menstruation and menopause discomforts; to cleanse infections

- **Related Womb Wellness: Mind Womb, Reproductive Womb –Eases anxiety of dis-order**
- **Application:** Add drops to baths and body lotions.
- **Note: Avoid Sage Oil: Pregnant women, babies, children and those with epilepsy.**

Affirmation:

I patiently and mindfully detoxify and rejuvenate my life. All is in Divine Order.

GATHER YOUR GEMSTONES

*G*emstones, often called "the bones of the Earth", are another wellness tools used by humans for thousands of years. As with all tools there are professionals who are trained to use them. I encourage you to seek their services in order to reap the optimum benefits of gemstone therapy. Meanwhile, as you empower yourself to take an active role in your own wellness, explore the world of precious and semi-precious stones.

Research shows a relationship between gemstone therapy and enhanced wellness to the inner being. Gemstone work focuses on your non-physical wombs: The Womb of the Heart (your emotions) and the Womb of your Mind (your thoughts). Listen to Voice of your inner Wombs, consider the properties of purification, amplification and balancing that are associated with gems.

Strategies for use of Gemstones

For personal hygiene and beauty:
- Wear jewelry –necklaces, bracelets, waist beads, earrings made from gemstones.

For your body:
- Place gemstones in and around your tub while you take your bath.

- Get a hot rock massage.

For your Wombs:
- Touch or hold the gemstones to your womb centers. Meditate for 5 to 15 minutes on empowerment and wellness.

For your space – home, office, car:
- Place a lose gemstones or a string of gemstones in place where you can see them and be reminded to stay strong and stand solid on your quest for your own wellness.

AMETHYST: Inspires meditation

- Related Womb Wellness: Mind Womb – Encourages mental strength

  Affirmation: *I release anger. I embrace the balance and beauty of my wellness.*

BLACK TOURMALINE: Disperses negativity

- Related Womb Wellness: Mind Womb, Heart Womb – Encourages positivity

   Affirmation: *I banish negative thoughts, emotions and diseases. I embrace the positivity of total Womb Wellness.*

BLOODSTONE: Supports strength an vitality of the body and solar plexus

- Related Womb Wellness: Mind Womb, Heart Womb – Encourages confidence

   Affirmation: *I can have total wellness. I am strong in all my parts from my womb core to my fingertips.*

CLEAR QUARTZ CRYSTAL: Supports clarity

- Related Womb Wellness: Mind Womb, Heart Womb – Encourages confidence to seek wellness

   Affirmation: *I can have total wellness. I am strong from my womb core to my fingertip.*

EMERALD (the birthing stone): Supports growth and transformation

- Related Womb Wellness: Mind Womb, Heart Womb, Reproductive Womb – Encourages growth

   Affirmation: *I deserve to be well. I consciously participate in my positive growth and development.*

LAPIS LAZULI: Relieves depression; supports idealism

- Related Womb Wellness: Mind Womb, Heart Womb – Encourages setting and reaching goals

  Affirmation: *My visions for my wellness are worthy. I deserve to have them. I can realize them.*

MALACHITE: Symbol of creativity and transformation

- Related Womb Wellness: Mind Womb, Heart Womb – Encourages balance and harmony

  Affirmation: *I am charging my inner wombs to support my ability for creativity, harmony and growth.*

MOONSTONE: Symbol of feminine and emotional energy

- Related Womb Wellness: Heart Womb – Soothes and calms emotions

  Affirmation: *I will not lose my temper and lose my serenity. I will seek calm and creative resolutions to conflicts. .*

ROSE QUARTZ: Supports clarity of the womb center

- Related Womb Wellness: Heart Womb – Restoration of compassion

  Affirmation: *I actively embrace achieving wellness for myself and all my relations.*

TURQUOISE: Absorbs negativity; purifies wounded wombs

- Related Womb Wellness: Mind Womb – Encourages restoration of wellness

  Affirmation: *My wombs can heal. I can celebrate my wellness*

'CAUSE, SISTERS, WE GOT ISSUES!

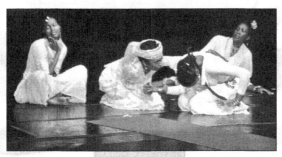

Actors telling the hurt away in a scene from: *The Womb Story*

*Y*ou have been reading through pages of strategies and may have already enjoyed using some of the tools for detoxification and restoration your wombs: Heart, Mind and Reproductive Center. The last pages of this portal are a guide to why and how to incorporate your relationships with your family and other relations into your new lifestyle of Natural Living. I have pointed out several womb issues and suggested how you can begin overcoming the damage and restoring your wellness.

In Portal Two, many women share their stories of trauma and triumph. Some of those stories are about relationships that caused a great deal of womb damage. Their stories show how womb issues that are buried later reveal themselves as *recycled* womb issues. They keep manifesting themselves in our relationships. Consciously and unconsciously we kept drawing to ourselves aspects of our hurt selves.

In many instances, womb issues, dramas and pains seem to go away only to resurface – deeper, more painful and more deadly as countless womb traumas and dramas. Womb issues left unattended and unhealed, return. Rape, incest, child abuse, abandonment, obesity are only some of the forms of womb damage that can and will continue, generation to generation if left unaddressed and unhealed.

Anger, war violence, greed, and jealousy are in the blood just as love, peace, and courage are in the blood. These events have made an impact on the human bloodline. Look into your bloodline as the blueprint of who you are and how you heal yourself Disease in your family history on the emotional and psychological levels does not have to keep you vibrating on a low frequency.

On the whole, humanity's bloodline has been poisoned, polluted. All of us on some level and in varied degrees are born to a family, a race, and/or an environment that brings profound challenge. Like a backpack of pain, we carry unresolved issues from childhood to adulthood. Unresolved issues, left in the memory of our bones, our heart, our womb, may be forgotten, but, is buried alive in our bloodlines getting stronger everyday. These issues build and become different forms of anger and pain.

We must explore our life lessons in order to overcome an angry vagina get beyond womb issues and achieve true lotus blossom essence (See PORTAL Four: REBIRTH). Womb healing and wellness takes time, thought and effort. Moving on physically does not mean that the pain stops immediately or the problem has been resolved. If we don't learn the lessons and work through our past pain, then we will have to continue relearning.

When will Womb Suffering end?

Listen to Voice of your Womb speak. She says:

"I will help to set you free from all our womb issues. Wrap your arms around yourself, around me and tell yourself and me how much you care for and love me. I will heal if you begin to care for us each and everyday. Forgive your parents if did not know how to love you. They were in their own pain. Forgive mates and other relationships that may have caused you pain, hurt and disease. They did not know how to love you. Maybe you will heal and one day, teach them through your wellness. Now, reach deep inside yourself for the greatest love there is and hold on tight to receive the love, guidance and protection from your Divine Mother-Father. We will be whole and well."

Womb wisdom is calling women from the four directions: the East, the North, the South, and the West. Align with the healer within. All of you who are seeking to end suffering from fibroids, PMS, heavy menses, vaginitis, cysts, sexual abuse, infertility, miscarriage, STDs, hot flashes, hysterectomy, prolapsed wombs, trauma and confusing sex for love.

Let us come into Womb Wisdom that we may globally and collectively heal our womb conditions and save lives by each woman beginning with her own sacred Womb Wellness. Use your tools and strategies.

You are not alone.

Maintain a Natural Living Lifestyle.

Form Circles with others who are ready to make changes for **Womb Wellness.**

Listen to the Voices of the Womb.

Meditate daily.

Write in your womb journal.

Believe your Womb Wellness can make a difference; the future of the world is in our wombs.

THE FUTURE OF THE WORLD IS IN OUR WOMBS

*I*n March, 2010 during International Women's Month, United Nations' Commission on the Status of Women sponsored a conference around the theme "Male Involvement in Promoting Human Rights for Women: Implications for Beijing + 15." The conference was held at the United Nations' Church Center, in New York. When I was given the opportunity to participate as a panelist, I shared the message of global womb wellness. As I said to the audience at the conference... **This is a call for a 28-Day Global Womb Detox and Rejuvenation for a Global Shift. It is a call** to create planetary womb wellness and to prevent further womb crimes – including the evidence of toxic spill-over and anger in the water, soil and air. We must begin to birth balanced, non-toxic children who will grow up and help to transform destructiveness into constructiveness. Women, if we plan to survive, we must collectively raise the vibration of our wombs. We must detoxify and rejuvenate.

Both women and men must cleanse. As women cleanse their wombs, men must cleanse their sperm and blood to change toxic, dis-eased, low-vibration fluids into purified, healthy fluids. Currently, toxic parents are giving birth to toxic babies who are addicted to drugs, alcohol, tobacco and non-live foods, as well as to negative thoughts and deeds. This is the time to encourage the restoration of purified men and women to produce life that will vibrate at a higher frequency of wellness.

The future of the world is in our wombs. Let us heal from the Angry Vagina and journey to Womb Wellness for global deliverance. A global womb detox will set the tone for women to wholistically prevent or heal from womb traumas ranging from fibroid tumors to venereal diseases. It is a means to minimize the occurrences of rape, incest and the other inhumane abuses manifested as dis-ease, greed, lust and war on global wombs.

The 28-Day Global Womb Detox and Rejuvenation should take place over 28 days to represent a lunar month cycle of new beginnings. As we cleanse we will work through womb issues one at a time. Starting at the roots, we need to investigate our early childhood so we can begin to forgive ourselves and the conditions causing angry vaginas. We must speak out; share in womb circles; write in our journals and fast. We need to include in our prayers the World Healing of Women whose human rights are challenged and the World Healing of Men who do not uphold human rights for their wives, daughters and mothers. Suppression of women's human rights ultimately destroys men as well. Liberation for some of us becomes liberation for all of us.

Our men cannot sit on the sidelines. Encourage your husband, brothers, sons and male family members to detox. Become a beacon of light to guide them to purge poisonous waste from their prostrate center which will improve their virility and sensitivity. Their healing will inspire them to continue to detox and purify.

DO NOT WAIT for anyone to fast and cleanse with you. Under no circumstances should you postpone your own healing. Collectively, hold the power inside our wombs for ultimate global liberation which cannot *"wombmanifest"* without our say and our action. Family and friends will become inspired by our example. They will follow in our footprints according to their level of awareness and readiness.

During the 28 days, purge your homes of physical and spiritual blockages to purity and wellness. Clean your work stations for greater clarity and balance on the job. Transform your kitchen into a healing laboratory. Feed your family life-giving foods and herbal tonics for cleansing body, mind and spirit. Focus on the men and women who are leaders in the political, spiritual and health sectors. Detoxified, they will be better-prepared to make well thought-out, enlightened decisions for themselves, their families and humanity.

Direct your family members to the hydrotherapy room (bathroom) three to four times a week. Hydrotherapy such as, herbal and salt baths, soaks, showers, sauna and steam baths, and Sweat Lodges promote wellness. These water therapies help to release mental and emotional pain, such as stress, anxiety, rage and depression. Encourage or assist family members to take enemas throughout the detox period order to flush toxic waste from the body and toxic attitudes from the mind and spirit.

Some of us may take one 28-day cycle to Heal Thyself, others may take longer. Often we remain in pain due to the lack of and/or inability to activate the knowledge to heal oneself. During the 28 days you will gain the knowledge and inspiration you need. If women collectively detox in harmony with the seasonal changes in their part of the globe, the entire planet will begin to vibrate to a level of purity that has not been witnessed since antiquity. During the 28-Day Global Womb Detox, we can become empowered by rising up with the sun –for, the early bird catches the blessings. We can offer forgiveness prayers; bathe; drink herbal tonics; eat organic foods and perform the Womb Yoga Dance (see Portal Five). We can begin to put an end to the madness that has damaged our wombs. We can envision a global rebirth to wellness.

Those who participate in the 28-Day Global Womb Detox are asked to consider the following levels of fasting:

Level I
Fast from negative thoughts, words and deeds; fast from viewing negativity on television and Internet

Level II
Fast from all cooked and processed foods. Instead, eat live foods.

Level III
Fast from solid foods. Instead, consume a liquid vegetable and fruit juices, herb teas and water.

If you are already on the path of Natural Living and have previously fasted you are are encouraged to perform at Level III. If you are unable to perform a total fast from solid food, then follow the Womb Wellness Diet to the best of your ability.

Optimum Detox and Purification. Some may be ready to declare 28 days of sexual abstinence. Embrace the purpose and benefits of conscious celibacy with love and gratitude. This will send a healing message to the entire planet. Closing down the gates of your "garden" will energize your spiritual attunement and atonement. It will diminish the negative consciousness that proliferates in the form of AIDS, incest, rape, domestic violence in the home, fibroid tumors and other attacks on the wombs of the world.

A sexual womb fast, or better said, "womb rest", would act as an atomic charge of world peace like nothing else can. Those who conceive after the 28-day Global Womb Detox will give birth to who are in a most elevated state of being, as was always intended for us.

To heal is to unblock energy, so that like an electrical current it will travel from one to another, allowing us to experience restoration of humanity *if* and as we purify. Human illnesses reflect adverse mental, physical and social and dietary imbalances. There are global environmental catastrophes – draught, volcanic eruptions, floods, earthquakes... The earth, like our wombs is speaking to us. We must listen. We, women and men, have the power to counteract the disastrous prophecies predicted by historical and contemporary visionaries and environmentalists. We can provide future generations with a wholesome legacy to the degree that we are willing to embrace our purification and wellness. A World Womb Detox can be a

Great Atonement to align us back to our natural lives. The 28-Day Global Womb Detox is not an overnight, quick–fix, it is a life path. Never has there been a greater need for a healing through a Global Womb Detox. Regardless of race, religion creed and dietary lifestyle, it is time to claim Liberation thru Purification.

Remember, within the **Lotus Seed**, nourished by the mud, growth can be realized. You can overcome an angry vagina and you can give birth to lotus visions and lotus children who are physically, mentally and spiritually balanced beings.

Be Well

DAILY WOMB WELLNESS CHECKLIST

Use the Daily Womb Wellness Checklist as your 28-Day guide.

	Sun	Mon	Tue	Wed	Thu	Fri	Sat
SUNRISE							
1. Reflection/meditation between 4 AM – 6 AM (light a candle; focus on womb centers – body mind and spirit)							
2. Pre-Breakfast: Kidney-Liver Flush - 1 Tbsp. Inner Colon Ease or olive oil in 1 warm water w/ juice of 1 lemon or lime							
3a. Daily Exercise: Power walk, Womb Yoga, Swim, etc.							
3b. The Pyramid (place legs at 45-degree angle against the bedpost as you lay flat in bed for 5–10 minutes 2X daily)							
3c. Squats (sit 5 minutes and breathe through the womb by contracting and releasing vaginal walls)							
4a. Liquid Breakfast: Fruit Juice with 2 Tbsp. GL*							
4b. Solid Breakfast: Fruit platter							
5. 3 tsp. Master Herbal Formula to 3 cups H_2O (Steeped overnight). Drink daily before 1 PM							

	Sun	Mon	Tue	Wed	Thu	Fri	Sat
MIDDAY							
6a. Liquid Lunch: 16 ozs. Green Juice with 2 Tbsp. GL*							
6b. Solid Lunch: steamed vegetables, green salad, vegetable protein							
7. Write in your journal at least once a day.							
8. Communicate daily with others who detoxing and purifying for mutual support							

	Sun	Mon	Tue	Wed	Thu	Fri	Sat
SUNSET							
9a. Liquid Dinner: 16 ozs. Green Juice 2 Tbsp. GL*							
9b. Solid Dinner: steamed vegetables, green salad with vegetable protein							
10. Listen to Empowerment CDs for re-enforcement; Consult with others in a Womb Wellness							
11. Colon wellness: Take herbal laxatives 1–3x per week; enemas 1–3x per week							

	Sun	Mon	Tue	Wed	Thu	Fri	Sat
12. Womb Wellness: Apply Clay Pack or Castor Oil Pack over the womb (see instructions); Drink Clay Tonic 3x weekly; Elevate legs at 450 angle, daily							
13. Full Body Bath morning or night. 1–4 lbs Epsom Salt or 1–2 lbs Dead Sea or Womb Wellness Ginger bath NO SALTS for those with blood pressure. Instead use 1 cup apple cider vinegar.							
14. Reflection/meditation before bedtime Focus on your womb centers – body, mind and spirit; Write in your journal.							

* GL= Green Life Formula

Drink 8 ozs. of warm H_2O during the liquid meal

Take a half an hour break between liquid and solid meal

PORTAL
Two

STORIES

Some of the stories were told to Queen Afua
and some are her own stories.

Some of the stories are from the voices of women
who could speak for themselves and some are from voices
that needed others to speak for them.

WARNING:

Some of the stories are extremely graphic and sensitive.
All of the stories are offered with love.

COMMON GROUND

Wombs bleeding, clotting, hearts weeping, wailing,
Hair done, face made-up, nails manicured
Dressed to the nines on the job
In the fields, in the factories, behind closed doors, behind the veil
We are on common ground.

Praying in the church, kneeling in the mosque, squatting in the sweat lodge,
Singing in the cathedral, meditating in the shrine, all the while our wombs are screaming.
We are on common ground.

From everywhere…deep inside, corporate workers banging on the glass ceiling
Blue-collar workers doing a day's work for a day's pay, city workers going by the rules,
Freedom fighters and entrepreneurs mothers and daughters suffer from the same conditions, passed
down through generations…

We drag around our womb stories,
from one relationship to the next in toxic womb conditions,
womb disregard, womb disrespect, broke-down, overused, exhausted wombs.
We're rising in the East,
We're facing the West,
Stretched out in the South,
Reaching for the North.
We are on common ground.

Womb stories, hidden, up under our dresses, lapas, shorts, and jeans
We wear our waist beads, pearls, diamonds, and moonstones
While tucked away behind our bladder in the privacy of our pubic center
… years of unresolved pain.
Trapped in our toxic reality womb stories
bursting through our veins reaching for relief.
We carry our pain in our purses, backpacks, and clutch bags
Can we find ourselves? Can we find our common ground?

All of us from the South of Common Ground
and the North of Deliverance
from the East of Womb Consciousness
from the West of Womb Wellness
We are reaching for our womb recovery.

We are women on Common Ground. We recognize one another.
We draw together, with our differences, and our sameness
to tell our stories.
Our tears pour from our wombs and fall onto the ground
—common ground--
The answers flow
onto the dirt,
onto the wood,
onto the marble,
onto the parquet floor
Our Common Ground becomes Sacred Ground
Where our medicine grows.
Out of our tears redemption flows,
Here on Common Ground.

Queen Afua/Spring 2009

Be courageous.

Form a womb circle or seek to join a womb circle.

Transverse through the mud and bloom into the lotus you are.

You deserve to heal yourself.

Join women in quilting circles and at dance class.

Circle with sisters in the beauty parlor or at the nail shop.

Chatting and texting you are a circle.

Talk to your mothers and cousins and godmothers.

Share wellness rituals at the spas and at seminars. Sister, Girlfriend, Daughter.

Six of you or twenty of you. Or one to one.

Each time you hear a story you are helping others

while you are helping yourself.

And, each time you tell your own story

you are getting closer to

your own womb restoration.

Listening to the Voice of the Womb is part of you healing yourself.

Listening to your stories and telling your stories

brings us all closer to Global Wellness.

No More...No More...No More...

I reflect on a gathering of women with the courage to share within a Womb Healing Circle.

I said: "Women, you are connected to your wombs by the forces of nature. Your womb is aware of her natural medicine; just ask and see. Go within, relax and breathe. Listen, what does your womb say and reveal to you?"

Within a Womb Healing Circle the women responded:

"My womb has had many visitations from a number of men over my life-time. She is tired and wants to rest."

Another woman jumped up...

"My womb wants to let go of these tumors, they are heavy and they hurt."

I asked the wombs to speak through the women and say what they wanted for them:

"I want her to stop cursing the men in her life and to pray for a light heart."

Another speaks...

"I want her to eat foods that are natural and I want her to fast from toxic foods."

And another...

"I love her. I want to be here for her. I am frightened 'cuz I am about to be cut out of her."

Woman after woman got up or just cried as their wombs spoke and they listened:

"I'm so full it hurts."

"I must share before I explode."

A woman is a little uptight and resistant about this womb talk business. She breathes in and opens her mouth to exhale. Her womb speaks in through her and to her in one word:

"Stop!"

There, in the back of the center, women began sharing their experiences. They wailed turmoil. Regardless of the story, we didn't judge one another, we were open and helpful. We were relieved to be able to connect to our wombs and share our womb stories. Finally, we were "unsilencing" the voices of our wombs.

In the front of the center, three men were purchasing products and my assistant was in my office. Although they could not hear the women's actual words, they all heard the wails from the circle of women. Each man had his own reaction. One leaned against the wall and bowed his head; the second leaned against the counter in a respectful silence. The third sat down and covered his eyes with his sunglasses. My assistant quietly wept. One of the women in the circle had come with her baby. Suddenly, she left the circle, went to the front of the center and asked my assistant to hold the child. As she walked back toward the healing circle she seemed to be on the edge. Then, letting go of something deep within, she began to wail. "No more! No more! No more!" Time stood still. When she finished releasing I had come to her side and asked her if she was ready to share her story. She said, "I am ready." I guided her toward the fifty-four women who cradled her back into their womb-healing circle. She held her head high, bravely. Slowly, she spoke of what happened to her from age 7 to 15. She told her story, in this safe place, to the ocean of women who poured love onto her wounded womb-soul. This woman spoke not only for herself but for many. Because of her courage to speak out, many women experienced healing that day. As she dried her tears she said, "I just want to let go and heal." In their own way, even the men purchasing products received a healing that day.

Queen Afua

Change Begins Within Me

I've constantly heard that "Change begins within." My cleansing work has opened the way for me to heal spiritually, emotionally, mentally, and physically. It's been about five years since I gave this testimony. Most importantly, I understand that my healing process truly is a journey. Sometimes the journey is lonely, sometimes confusing, and often times scary and grueling. But, it has sweet rewards. I have gained access to the ultimate VIP pass to my Inner Self, my Higher Self, and more that are just waiting for me to blossom and to shine like the moonlight that I am.

My womb's pains and traumas have a story of their own –a story that when shared will turn into gold. I've learned that there's value in sharing to help unlock the pain. When I shared in a safe and constructive environment, I was supported, strengthened, and freed. My testimony gave encouragement to others. I am grateful to God, to my Higher Self, and to those who shared with me. They opened my ears and my soul. I am grateful to Queen Afua for her steadfastness on her journey and for her continuous service as a loving, spiritual mid-wife to thousands of women. She serves as a stellar example of self-love and care. May all of us stay blessed.

SW TaMerRa Het-heru
(La Tayla Monique Palmer-Lewis)

Missing Link

Dear Queen Afua,

As I told you when we met, I had been on a twenty-two year quest for inner freedom. My quest guided me to you and the Sacred Woman classes. I told you I wanted to embrace a natural living lifestyle. I needed a deep cleansing and hoped to receive the maximum healing possible. During the eleven week training period I worked on many personal issues which included fibroids and vaginal cysts.

After I completed the Sacred Woman Rites of Passage Training, I continued to work on myself. In conjunction with my physical exercises, I created a regiment of juicing my vegetables, drinking wheat grass, taking enemas and taking Epsom salts and sea salt baths. The whole process lasted six months. I continued to seek the medical diagnosis of my family doctor and followed his instructions. You encouraged me to keep notes to document my progress. I am proud to claim and testify that I became completely fibroid free and the cysts have split into pieces. I continued to eat raw foods, juice my vegetables and I drink a lot of water.

I have been following the Natural Living program. When I went to my doctor for another diagnosis of the fibroids and vaginal cysts we were both amazed to discover that there was no evidence of the pre-existing condition. I am overjoyed! All the work I have been doing is paying off. Slowly, I am learning how to live naturally and I am growing into my divine self. I am taking really good care of myself and I am happy to do it. I'm having a blast! Queen Afua, thank you from the bottom of my heart. I will continue using what I learned from you. It was the missing link in my life-long journey for wellness.

Submitted with Blessings and Love and Gratitude

Testimony of a Miracle

I have known Queen Afua since she was 9 years old. I was her day camp counselor. We lost contact for many years. Through my god-brother, we reconnected. I had just had a miscarriage. I did not know I had fibroid tumors until I had the miscarriage. I had been a devotee of medical doctors. After I was released from the hospital, I went to see Queen Afua. I was bleeding profusely. She immediately gave me a colonic and herbs. Once I started to drink the goldenrod tea—the bleeding stopped. Queen Afua suggested that I do a 21-Day fast. I strongly resisted. I wanted a pork sandwich. However, on New Year's Day 1985, I began a 21-Day fast. I lost a great deal of weight. I could feel the fibroids moving around in my womb. I had been told that I could never have a child and I should have a hysterectomy. I was determined to have a child. My biological clock was ticking. Fasting and cleansing were the beginning of a miracle for me. After months of fasting and cleansing, I conceived my precious daughter. In 1986, exactly one year after I began my cleansing, I gave birth to my daughter, Yemonjah Sango. As a result of raising my daughter in a natural, toxin-free way, she has known good health from birth.

Submitted by Gail Togan

A Natural Miracle

I was plagued with fibroid tumors and the related complications for years. I was experiencing a 22-day monthly period of heavy bleeding. I was hemorrhaging. Within less than 6 months of fasting, juicing and eating properly, my tumors have completely gone. After fasting and cleansing my period went down to a four-day flow. No more pain. No more clotting. No more PMS. What a relief! Today it feels so good to be alive and healthy. Thus, the miracle of me, Pansy Kiffin. Queen Afua has been an inspiration and a blessing in my life. Thank you and lots of love.

Womb Issues

I began to heal my life on the spiritual, mental and physical levels. I began to understand about karmic debts I owed due to my actions. I was at war within myself, full of greed, anger and fear. Trapped in "hell", I sabotaged every potentially beautiful relationship. By the age of 16 I had contracted the herpes virus. Keeping this a secret was suffocating me. Then I was diagnosed with endometriosis, fibroid tumors and ovarian cysts. The doctor said these conditions would eventually cause cancer and infertility. He suggested surgery, but he said he could not guarantee that I would ever be totally cured.

I was ready to take on my own healing and I sought out Queen Afua to guide me. She gave me a nutritional vegetarian diet to follow and instructed me to take enemas daily, drink plenty of chlorophyll and use clay packs. I took a stand and followed Queen's guide as if I was possessed. I become responsible for the unhappiness in my life. Throughout this love journey, I realized that I was the mirror of my environment. My life was so toxic-filled with deception and various manipulations, that I was ashamed of myself. I told people of my past and present about my herpes virus. I chanted and prayed for their forgiveness and stared to live a life of compassion, patience, trust and integrity. A new beginning unveiled...a miracle.

My womb started to forgive me and began to heal. I returned to my medical doctor and was diagnosed as being free of fibroids, cysts and endometriosis. The herpes outbreaks had stopped! Also, I no longer suffered with the miseries associated with menstruation.

Within 3 months I was pregnant. I had no sickness of any kind. In 2001, my beloved son was born with a birth weight of 9 lbs, 14oz. He is vibrant and full of life and has an extremely calm demeanor. He is a gift of life. I feel blessed. Through the birth of my son I have shifted to be more responsible for my health and life. Since my womb healing, my husband and I are living more and more in health and harmony. I am forever grateful for my karma guiding me to my Miracle Earth Mother, Queen Afua. She helped to awaken me to love my life.

Nylah

Positive Turn

In 1982, I was diagnosed with pelvic inflammatory disease (PID). During my hospital stay I was also diagnosed with fibroid tumors. These tumors caused no problems until 1989 when the gynecologist immediately suggested that I get a complete hysterectomy. I was a 30 year-old single mother of one child. I was hoping to get married and have more children.

Between 1988 and 1993, I enlisted the advice of four more doctors. The last doctor apologized to me for the pain and suffering I had endured throughout my search for alternatives to a hysterectomy. During this time, I was trying several wholistic approaches, which I am confident kept the fibroids "under control." Nonetheless, the fibroids grew to the size of a 24 week old fetus. In 1994, I opted to have an allopathic surgeon remove the fibroids laser myomectomy surgery. Over 200 tumors were removed during this surgery.

In the thirteen years, from 1974 to 1987, I was involved in five destructive relationships which left me with low self-esteem. I was harboring anger and resentment in my body and in my soul. I felt unable to do any better and feared being without a man in my life. Between March 1987 and December 1989, I lived a holistic lifestyle. I prayed, fasted and said daily affirmations. I gave up dating and sex so that I could focus on getting my life back in order. In turn for my sacrifices and cleansing, I was blessed with a husband (we got married in 1992) who supports my endeavors wholeheartedly. My husband does not pass any judgment on me for who and what I was in the past. He loves me for *who and what* I have become.

Bedside Manner

I was 39 years old. Single. Sexually active with one partner. As a teacher and grad school student, I had an aerobic-level schedule. My figure was a tad "thick", as they say. I treated my voluptuous bosom to fabulous bras. No mammograms yet. My menstrual periods and Pap exams were "normal." I planned to get pregnant before the BIG 4-0. My internal clock was ticking.

On the anniversary of my grandmother's death, I was thinking about the women in our family. Sturdy stock. Both grandmothers had been single moms in the

1930s. I could do this. I had a reliable income, a Master's Degree, two passports-worth of travel; family support. It was almost the 1990s. Suddenly, sprinting through a maze of rambunctious eighth-graders, I felt an unbelievable pain in my belly; like a mule had just kicked me. The pain doubled me in half, like nothing since teenage cramps. It took my breath and made me stagger. Was I having a heart attack? In my *womb*? My co-worker got me some water and made me an appointment with her gynecologist for later that day. She promised that he was "the best" and would fix me up.

Dr. "The Best" pissed me off. Throughout an unnecessarily painful pelvic exam, he had a conversation (about horror movies) with the nurse; but no conversation with me. **NONE!** Gloves on...speculum in...poke, prod, poke...speculum out...gloves off...doctor gone. The nurse told me to get dressed.

I was shaking when Dr. "Horror Movie" said, "You have fibroid tumors." I thought, *Tumors... cancer. Nobody in our family ever had cancer. OK, take them out...take medicine...even chemo. Get fixed. Get pregnant.* The "baby-time" ticking was Big Ben loud. I channeled my grandmothers for strength. "Doctor, what is the prognosis for cure and then conceiving a child?" Yes, *dammit!* My arrogance was good genes, good health insurance and a good vocabulary. He was stunned, "You need a uterus to conceive in, young lady. You won't have one after your hysterectomy. See my nurse for a surgery date." I like to recall that I left without paying Dr. "Horrible Bedside Manner" for the pain during the exam and his nonchalant plans to murder my womb. I cried all the way from Harlem to Brooklyn.

Later, my home-girl, a nurse-midwife, explained to me that most fibroids are not cancerous. Another sister-girlfriend directed me to Dr. Martin Greenberg, who is a legendary pioneer of the laser myomectomy procedure (fibroid removal *without* uterus removal). This *real* Dr. "The Best" always wore a button with the word HYSTERECTOMY in black letters crossed out by a big red "X."

Two years later, after I had suffered a miscarriage—that's another story—Dr. Greenberg, removed over one hundred fibroids from my uterus. He left my womb in tact, and encouraged me to, "Try again." I was 41 years old and Dr. Greenberg believed it wasn't too late.

Titi

Womb Removed

E-mails:

Dear G,

This happened back in 1994 and I have never been able to put words to my experience.

I had no idea my doctor was going to take the picture but the moment I saw it I was in shock.

My womb on the table. Taken out of me. It looked like a frightened /sad face.

I explained that to Queen.

K

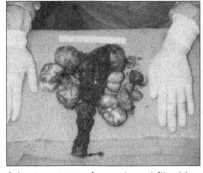

A hysterectomy. A womb and fibroids removed.

Dear K,

The book I am working on for Queen is titled: Overcoming an Angry Vagina: Journey to Womb Wellness. I've taken the liberty to send you my story as you have already generously shared yours.

In the name of the sisters who may benefit from either or both, may Spirit and the ancestors continue to guide and protect all of us.

Love and green from Brooklyn,
G

Dear G,

Powerful title....personal stories...wish I would have sought out a book that might have triggered me to think in alternative ways. I was about to loose my health insurance and felt backed against the wall. Glad you had people around you at the right time and more importantly, you listened. Wow 100 fibroid tumors...our bodies certainly do struggle waiting for us to claim health. Continued economic, physical and spiritual prosperity on your journey towards the publication of Overcoming an Angry Vagina.

Peace - Love - Blessings,
K

Queen Afua tells the story of a woman's ...

Decision

It was the third week of February 1996. On Friday night I gave a Liberation Thru Purification presentation at a New Jersey Baptist Church. The next morning I took a plane out of town to lecture at Ohio State University. Sunday I gave a keynote speech at Union DC 37 in Manhattan –after having attended an African spiritual service in Brooklyn. I was on a "Wellness Roll" spreading the Heal Thyself message throughout the land. Everything was going according to Divine Plan.

The following Thursday I gave a presentation at the NYC Transit Authority in a conference room filled with wholistically conscious women and men. After the presentation I was stopped in my tracks by a woman with her mind fully made up. She said, "Queen Afua, I've decided to remove my womb." I took a deep breath and let it out slowly. She went on to say, "I'm just tired of the pain and the bleeding and the tumors." My reply to her was, "Then prepare, Sister! Prepare your body and womb by drinking large amounts of live juices. Eat fresh and dried herbs and eat only natural foods as you place your life in the hands of the Divine. Maintain constant contact with the Creator through meditation and prayer, then, when you come out of surgery your body temple will recover in less time than surgeons suggest." With a great deal of love and an inner smile, I said "Peace be upon you and your womb." We hugged and then went our separate ways.

In my travels, I sometimes think of this woman and send her a prayer. My prayer for her is that the Divinity within her will evoke a life of serenity. I pray that after her surgery, she will remain whole and intact for the rest of her life's journey. I also pray that one day I will look up in a womb circle and see her there praying with her sisters for world womb deliverance

No Intention

Dearest Queen Afua:

In December 2002, I went to my GYN doctor because I thought I was pregnant; I was six weeks late. On the sonogram, my doctor noticed my right ovary was enlarged. I was diagnosed with a dermoid ovarian tumor* and several cysts. I was told that my only option was to have them removed. There was a great risk of permanent damage to my ovaries. The second doctor I spoke to was a Chief of GYN-Oncology. I was warned that a hysterectomy might be necessary to avoid cancer. He requested me to sign papers authorizing him to remove my womb if necessary while I was still under anesthesia. I thought, "Lose my womb—Never!" So, I went for second and third opinions. The doctors all agreed, "Have the surgery." "Have a hysterectomy." "Do not waste time with a holistic approach. The tumor will only get bigger and worse."

"You already have a child. You can live without a womb, Go ahead—take it out."

I was surprised at the doctors' blasé and nonchalant attitude. They did not understand that I had no intention of Giving Up My Womb! My womb is special and beautiful to me. The doctors were pressing me to have the surgery soon. I was terrified, anxious, depressed and stressed out. Hopeless, I scheduled the surgery thinking, "The doctors must be right as they are all saying the same thing."

Several sister-girlfriends urged me not to feel hopeless. One woman, a precious rock, comforted me during my sleepless nights. She advised, motivated, and directed me to take charge of my life. She encouraged me to investigate more and not to give in to the doctors' pressures. This woman directed me back to you. You recharged me and referred me to a "regular" physician who understands the importance of natural healing. I took herbs. I followed a Natural Living plan for thirty days before. A wonderful friend helped me to juice wheatgrass. My devoted family reminded me that I am Divine Light and I Can Heal Myself. Thirty days later the tumor is gone. My ovaries are normal and my womb is intact. The doctors were WRONG! So, I thank you from my soul. My womb thanks you for your dedication to helping so many people to heal themselves. The work you do is beautiful and so necessary. I will stay on the Natural Living path. You have my deepest appreciation.

Jessica HetHeru Bate

PS: One year later Jessica gave birth to a healthy baby girl.

* A dermoid cyst contains the same tissue as skin, fat, bone, hair, or cartilage; may become inflamed or cause ovarian twisting.

Save Me from the Drama

I'm over 55 years. I look young for my age, so they say. I haven't been beaten up by womb drama. I am sure this has given me my "womb grace." I've been eating wholistically since I was a teenager. I don't bleed heavy and I don't seem to attract womb trauma and womb dis-ease. I had a mate early on. He was a good man, but we just weren't meant to be. I never got pregnant 'cause I used natural birth control; unlike many of my friends who got pregnant out of wedlock. They had several abortions causing them to cry "a river of tears." I feel blessed to be a woman. My Mommy and Daddy raised me with love so I didn't carry over any negative baggage from my youth to my adulthood. I learned from my parents that people are people, so I keep my heart light. Witnessing all my sisters and hearing their womb stories, I decided early on to avoid the womb drama. I decided to wait to be sexually intimate for when I am married no matter how long it took. I worked at saving myself from the "drama."

Lady Prema (Queen Afua's lifelong friend)

Purged

When negative experiences with men remain trapped in women's minds it is a sign that they are also holding negative pain in their wombs. Queen Afua asks a group of women in a womb circle to call out the man or men who they were still holding onto after the relationship was over. She whispers encouragement for them to share their womb stories and purge themselves of the negativity so that they may be restored to their original beauty. The women are lying on the floor. One by one they let down their defenses and began to release the pain associated with the men. They call out the names: *"Bobby." "Paul." "Jim." "Kwami." "Joseph." "Neil."* The negativity and pain begin to fly out of the wombs-souls of the women. The room vibrates with the collective womb detox exercise. There begins to be calmness after the storm.

One woman sits against the wall wrapped up in her body like a knot. She says, "I won't call out his name, I hate him so... he was cruel... he hurt me so bad." A tear rolls down her cheek. Queen Afua puts her hand under the woman's chin and catches the tear in her palm. "This tear is the hurt, this tear is the essence of who is lodged in your womb", Queen says. "Cry and drain him out of your womb. Let him go so you can recover. Continue to weep and release and learn from the lessons that brought such pain. Queen hugs the woman who weeps her release.

ANGRY VAGINA DRIVE-BY STORIES

Is It Sex? Is It Love?

He beat me down and then he apologized with HOT SEX. I know he really does love me. "It won't happen again", he promised. But then, it happens again and again.......and again. If I stay in this relationship, I will be a member of "The Battered Wives Club." Makeup sex is abusive behavior. The lovin' act is violent. My husband is a predator. He communicates with me through violent sex. This is not love. He does not love me. Maybe I do not love myself. We communicate with arguments and yelling and hitting and crying, just me crying and then sex-ing. I gotta get off this merry-go-round and run for my life. I need to fix my life. I need to love myself. I need to fix this mess.

Hit and Run

I met this wonderful man. He was everything I always wanted. I finally struck gold after so many duds. Even the sex is hot. He told me and showed me in many ways that he loved me. Everything was not perfect, but that's life. He wouldn't give me his cell number. He always came over to my place; I was never invited to his. When I would bring it up he would find a way to change the sub-ject. I told him all about my life but I knew very little about his and his back-ground or his family. He told me I was the love of his life.

When I started feeling nauseous and throwing up I went to my doctor. I was pregnant. I was in shock but it was okay because I knew my man loved me. I sat my man down a few days after I found out that we were having a baby. He said, "I never told you I wanted a baby. I'm not trying to be a father." This man of my life, my gold turned into tin when he said, "So, what are you gonna' do?" After we argued he gave me a check for an abortion. I never saw him again.

Why did I attract such a horrible scene? Will I ever get over it?

Bip-Bam ThankYou, Ma'am

I need a man, but I really want a husband. I keep meeting these one-night stands. I find men in the club, on vacation, on the run. Sex is our connection. I really want more. The way he looks at me, touches my face so gently, speaks to me so sincerely... my heart opens, I stop thinking. In no time I let him enter my...special love spot. I believe this is the one. It has to be.

The next day I reach out for him, my sweet lover, but he doesn't reach out to me. Days go by and the phone is dead. I cry the endless tears. I realize, once again I am: a Bip Bam, Thank you, Ma'am Woman. Why is this the only kind of men I get?

The Down Low Saga

I was having unprotected sex with strangers. They never stayed long. "I just want a man." Everyday I chant, "I just want a man... I just want a man... I just want a man..." I only feel fulfilled when somebody is deep inside of me. Well, I got a man and this time he gave me more than sex. I found out later that I had had sex with a *down low brother*. He was secretly having sex with men and then with women! He had gotten AIDS and was spreading it around. Now, I've been infected. AIDS dropped off right into my....*you know*... It was like I had given that man permission to destroy me!! What am I supposed to do, now?

Keeping Myself Sacred

While on the journey of my Sacred Woman training I noticed I was becoming illuminated and attracting suitors like bees to honey. Keeping my womb sacred was challenging. Men saw the Divine in me...started to call me, "Goddess" and "Queen." They said they had to "have" me. I told them, "You must fast and cleanse to get rid of your toxicity...then and only then can we think about consummating our relationship." They could not believe me. Each one responded, "I'm not changing my diet just to be with you." or "I am meat! I come from meat."

"Too bad, it's your loss," I said. You see, there is no other way. My sisters and I have concluded that even a condom can not keep out the poisons. There is no choice for me but to continue on my path and stay clean from toxic foods and toxic men. As I wait for my Sacred Man who is also on the path to healing himself, I will surround myself with Sacred Women who support my Womb Wellness and their own. I know he's out there.

Lotus Blossom Womb Sharing from a Sacred Woman

Natural Child Birth

I was 36 years old and two months pregnant. I had two children delivered by C-section because of my high blood pressure. My father had died of cancer and diabetes. My mother and grandmother had wellness issues. I did no want to suffer this way. I absolutely did not want to have another C-section. I sought consultation with Queen Afua to help me help myself.

I decided to let go of major stress by leaving my job. I changed my diet drastically by eliminating meat and adding plenty of natural foods and teas. I lost weight I had gained from eating in a toxic way. Spiritually, I chanted and dedicated myself to having a healthy pregnancy and natural delivery. Queen Afua recommended herbal baths, the Dance of the Womb exercises, staying peaceful and balanced and getting plenty of rest. My husband and I found a midwife, "M", who would assist us with natural birth in a hospital birthing center. "M" finally found a doctor willing to help us despite my history of complications. June 25 th was my due date.

On July 7th, I was two weeks overdue. The doctor advised me to come in two days later for a non-stress test. He said he might have to "take the baby." My husband and I maintained our position against a C-section delivery. "M" promised to support us. That evening I felt a sharp pain I didn't recognize because I had never experienced labor before. For the next six hours I tried to prepare myself holistically with castor oil, herbal teas, showers and an enema. The contractions got stronger. I knew I would not need the non-stress test because my baby was coming that night.

At 1:00 AM hardly anyone was on the road or in the emergency room. The way was open for us. In the labor room, when my water broke, neither the doctor nor the midwife was there. Finally, "M" arrived. She soothed everyone with her calm spirit. S"M"he encouraged me to breathe deeply and to call for my baby to come forth. I made a soft family *hissing* sound and our son was born on the fourth push. It was beautiful. They put our son on my chest and my husband cut the umbilical cord. His name, Azikiwea, is Nigerian for "healthy, forceful, strong, and virtuous." My pregnancy had been all those things and that is the way we want him to tackle the world. I had been totally vegan and frequently when I had taken a few drops of Queen Afua's Breath of Spring and had done my fire breaths, I had felt Azikiwea moving vigorously inside me.

At 8 pounds, 10 ounces, he was the biggest of all of my children. He was not born crying, nor was he covered with mucus. His first breaths were not congested. He came forth clean and clear with his eyes wide open. Four hours later Azikiwea was fully alert, not lethargic. I had no medication, no monitors, no doctors. I had no back pains, no high blood pressure, no swollen ankles, and NO C-SECTION! I felt so alive.

A pleasant surprise was that one of the nurses had studied holistic strategies with Queen Afua like I had. It was a good sign. Now a devout believer in the Natural Way, I am pleased I sought Queen Afua's help and advice. Azikiwea is a well and peaceful child.

Sister Roseanne TaUrt

The Creator Lifts Me UP

September 18th, 1994. On this day, the anniversary of my birth, I write this testimonial in the hope of sharing life and hope. Over a year ago, I was told that I fibroid tumors. I panicked because I know that these "growing" things were detrimental to my happiness in this life. They might prevent my ability to bring life. At first, I was frightened and then I became furious. What are fibroids? I was not born with them and I certainly will not leave with them. I embarked on a quest for knowledge. My mission has been fulfilled. The Divine Creator led me to read *Heal Thyself for Health and Longevity* by Queen Afua and I commenced to following her program. Through fasting, prayer and a life of strict discipline, I rid myself of fibroid tumors which amazed my doctors and proved that I could heal myself. Today, I am blessedly 51/2 months pregnant. My diet has not changed backwards. I will not eat flesh foods or dead foods—and neither will my child. After all, how can I enrich life with death?

In my pregnancy I have not experienced the "regular" symptoms of pregnancy. No morning sickness, no enormous weight gain, no fatigue, no swollen feet, no hair loss, no blotchy skin and no evilness of spirit. I look and feel beautiful! During this time, I have met countless women who also live with the horror of fibroids, cancer and/or cysts. These ailments seem to have become commonplace among us!

They don't have to be!

They must not be!

They will not be!

My sisters, heal yourselves, and your body temples. We are the carriers of life. Let nothing keep us from our divine mission. May you find joy through cleansing as I have.

Submitted from Oluwa Yemisi Adewkumi

Healing Journey

Before embarking upon my womb healing journey, the solution to my menses agony was 800 milligrams of ibuprofen to silence my womb cries. I knew my womb tantrums were due to my diet. During my late teenage years, I managed to rid myself of eczema breakouts and heavy mucus congestion by eliminating milk and adopting a moderate vegetarian lifestyle. However, I was not working at optimal level to heal myself. Consequently, I was vulnerable to acne, back pains, emotional imbalance, nausea and menstrual fatigue. If would get so bad, that if I did not take painkillers I would throw up all my food. Almost anything would make me cry. Curled up in fetus-position, I suffered an assortment of imbalanced emotional thoughts about forgiveness, irreconcilable differences and anger. My womb was fighting like a warrior to survive; she also mourned that I ate "dead" food. Beyond hygiene upkeep, our bond was in discord. In my busy lifestyle, I gave so much of myself without taking adequate time to replenish; I would quickly get burnt out. I operated on "one leg" and a prayer to accomplish my duties and my goals.

I bought *Sacred Woman and Heal Thyself* and applied some methods but mostly blocked fully changing my lifestyle. I was not patient enough. The one thing that I was consistent with was prayer. Prayer led me to Brooklyn where I documented the "City of Wellness" event held at the Queen Afua Wellness Institute. I reconnected to my knowledge about wellness when Queen Afua said, "You are not supposed to suffer and experience heavy bleeding; here is what you need to do…!"

Is have my 21-Day Fast Kit from Queen Afua and I have been healing at a rapid rate. I must confess, I did slip by eating a toxic food and was reminded of my mistake with the almost unbearable period pains I have ever known. This was the reaction of an uncompromising and angry vagina. I refused to reach for medication and went through the healing process by continuing my fasting program. After one day, my womb released her iron grip of retaliation. I was pain free! I began to fully understand bonding with my womb and how all my actions and thoughts correlate to her well-being.

I hope sharing this covenant I have chosen for myself inspires many to heal thyself and all their relations. With among the highest frequency of gratitude, I am thankful for Queen Afua's unwavering passion for healing and uplifting the people.

LOVE & LIGHT,
D. H.

Warning:
Graphic material on clitoridectomy:

Rite of Passage

There is a womb war going on. Wombs are being killed, bombed, mutilated, violated...CUT AWAY. I do not like what has happened to me, my mothers and my sisters....

I was 13 years of age when my womb and my labia were cut away. My vagina was sewn together by women of my village who had comforted me throughout most of my life. I trusted them.Since this was done to me, something deep inside me shut down and died. My womaness, my power and my beauty have been cut away. I can't speak out. I can't speak out. My womb hurts, but I cannot speak out. I must understand, this is tradition for my people. It is a Rite of Passage. If I speak out I will lose my family. I will not get a husband to protect me. If I dare to speak out there will be a great division and a great loss. I'm silenced by my own people. I am enraged. But I must stay quiet. I do not have the power to change anything. I have to keep accepting this act again and again. My daughters and my daughters' daughters and all of us will be cut. Years later, the pain of a sharp knife cutting out my clitoris is still fresh in my mind; but what could I do? It was done to all the women by the elder women of my village. Our mothers and aunties watch on and on and on...

I wish to know when it will come to an end.

Warning:
Graphic material on incest:

Help Me

"Hi, Daddy...No, Daddy...I don't want to play that game again."
"No, Daddy...You are hurting me...
"Mommy, help me."

I'm Mad As Hell

I have experienced abuse, violation, love lost and deception within my womb-soul-self. I hated my father. When he wasn't sexing me he gave me nice things and helped me complete my homework. On Saturdays, he took me to dance and piano lessons. This confused me because I wanted to hate my father for forcing sex on me and stealing my innocence.

Now that I am a woman, I keep asking myself, "How could my father hurt me like that over and over again? How can I trust any man?"

They told me that it happened generation to generation. His father had committed incest with his daughters, my aunts. Sometimes I think that the poison in my family goes way back to slavery. Maybe six or seven generations back. I think it takes a lot of hate for a father to rape his daughters. Fathers sexed their daughters, uncles sexed their nieces, and even brothers sexed their sisters.

My father raped me. How could he do that? Why did he do that to me? I feel a lot of pain. I'm mad as hell.

Bloodline

Recently the community was made aware of a father having sex with his four daughters from ages 6 to 14. A household was filled with endless shouts of, "Daddy, stop you are hurting me! Please, stop!" How did this abusive behavior become the norm of this family's existence? How did night cries, screaming and tears become the accepted family dialogue? How far back and how deep does the damage go? What is to become of these daughters? When they grow into women will they bear children? Will they have mates? Will their offspring become part of another generation of incest, pain and abuse? How many damaged wombs and hearts and sprits have been passed through the bloodline from generation to generation to generation?

83

VOICELESS

Around the world, throughout the history of humankind,
one group overpowered another.
Those who overpowered were called the "masters";
those who lost their personal freedom were called the "slaves."

One result of enslavement is
that females — adults and children — are forced
to have sex against their will; raped.

The space below on this page has been left blank in honor of the
thousands upon thousands of stories that never got told; never got written.
This space is for the voices of the daughters, nieces, dancers, seamstresses,
teachers, famers, queens, mothers, artists, girls, sisters, grandmothers,
princesses, women…Their stories continue in the wombs of all of us.

GLOBAL VOICES OF ANGRY VAGINAS

Voices of Angry Vaginas in Morocco: Moroccan women and several human rights organization like the Moroccan Human Rights Association have asked for an inquiry into forced prostitution of young women which has become very common in Morocco.

Voices of Angry Vaginas in Nigeria: Reproductive health issues have glaring disparities within West Africa. Countless Nigerian women are subjugated to serious human rights violations—especially with regard to their reproductive health choices and care. Many unofficial reports of rape, genital mutilations and forced prostitution remain unaddressed by world leaders.

Voices of Angry Vaginas in South Africa: Health options for women in South Africa are secondary to genocide activity in this region. Women of all ages are victims of rape, prostitution, AIDS, STDs and other human rights violations that are not exposed in most international reports. Corrective action is needed.

Voices of Angry Vaginas in Afghanistan: Hundreds of women have been killed because male relatives are on the mission of protecting "family honor." "Honor killings" are murders of females committed by male relatives, based only on suspicion that the female has been sexually promiscuous; even if the woman was raped. This total disregard of the woman's life allows men to be "heroes" and remain unpunished for murder.

Voices of Angry Vaginas in China: Due to China's long history of national privacy, the rapes and dehumanization of Chinese women has been internationally unavailable. Little or no corrective action has been taken regarding the number of rapes "informally reported" to the authorities.

Voices of Angry Vaginas in Thailand: Most poor women are forced into prostitution to support themselves and their families. Thousands of Thai women, especially young girls are regularly subjected to gang rape, beatings and domestic violence. There is a tremendous loss of life as a result of these acts that generally are unpunished by Thai authorities.

Voices of Angry Vaginas in Mexico: Domestic violence and sexual harassment in the workplace are common and customary in most economically underdeveloped countries. According to reports from several trade union officials, women workers are harassed regularly in Mexico.

Voices of Angry Vaginas in Guatemala: Guatemala has one of the worst human rights records in the Western Hemisphere. Over 90% of Guatemalan human rights violations are committed upon people under the control of state security. Young women are regularly subjected to gang rape.

Voices of Angry Vaginas in the Caribbean: Throughout the English, French and Spanish speaking islands of the Caribbean, women experience serious womb diseases and imbalances. Reports on the increase of sexual violence (rape, mutilation and assault), fibroid tumors and hysterectomies and cervical and uterine cancers have yet to be properly documented as women's health issues are heavily guarded in these world-renowned tropical "paradises."

Voices of Angry Vaginas in Australia: The most severe poverty in Australia exists in the Aboriginal and Torres Strait Islander communities; this is about half a million Australians. Over 200 years of racism and disenfranchisement have left Indigenous Australians with the lowest levels of education, the highest levels of unemployment, the poorest health and unthinkable housing conditions.

Voices of Angry Vaginas in Canada: In Canada, a woman is sexually assaulted every 6 minutes. 1 in 3 women in Canada will be sexually assaulted at some time in their lives. 1 in 4 women are at the risk of rape or attempted rape in her lifetime. 1 in 8 women will be sexually assaulted while attending college or university.

Men and women in support of Womb Wellness,
we must Rebirth the Earth.
We must overcome the Angry Vagina.

THE CHANGE

At age fifty I went into **menopause**. It was the summer of 2002, and I thought my hot flashes were due to environmental heat that caused me to sweat. Menopause caught me off guard. It was a shock. I thought, not me! I'm wholistic. This can't be happening to me. I wanted to deny its existence; but the sweats could not be denied. I was making a hormonal shift. It took me a year to adjust physically and psychologically to THE CHANGE. I was frightened. For the first time I thought, this is what old age must feel like. *But I don't believe in old age!* I believe that as long as you take really great care of yourself you will avoid the old age symptoms and be vital throughout your life. My belief was almost **shattered!** If I wanted to enjoy my maturity I had to *really* put my health first and be even more consistent with my wellness than ever before. So I went deep into myself. I had put two adult children through college and helped the third with his career development. I had grown two businesses—*Heal Thyself, TM, Inc.* and *Sacred Woman, Inc.* Surely, I could do this!

I am embracing my new stage of life wholistically through the fears, the tears and the resistance to ask for the support of my sisters about this rite of passage, menopause. Since then I have strapped on my tools of wellness – including sister circle love. Menopause will not "drive" me into the ground. Instead I intend to "ride" this eldership piece powerfully and to arrive at the threshold of many more rites of passage fully charged.

P.S. I can still stand on my head!

Queen Afua

21ST CENTURY TESTIMONIALS

*T*he stories in this portal are evidence that women and their families have been receiving wellness consultations and instructions from Queen Afua for nearly three decades. Groundwork for this text, the documentation of Queen's ongoing Womb Wellness work, was laid in the mid-1990s. The following are excerpts from stories of rejuvenation and testimonials to Queen Afua that continue into the new millennium.

I am the mother of three sons...my family and community relationships require thought and energy. Drinking the Heal Thyself Formula II you created is like a retreat for me. I love the way it makes me feel energetic and focused...

Thank you, Princess Ameenah

The Queen Afua teachings work as a constant and timely reminder of wellness awareness...wonderful and refreshing for the body and soul; the reset button for the mind.

Kris Gounden – Activist

Queen Afua taught me "that light cast out dark... negative power is disguised as mental illness, physical illness, spiritual illness..." I have carried this message through my thoughts, deeds and actions...Seventeen years later I continue to be strengthened by her wisdom and resolve...I applaud her as one of my greatest teachers and inspirations.

Eternal light, Asherah formerly known as Arlene Xavier

A few years ago, a Mammogram displayed that I had a cyst on my left breast. I followed the steps Queen Afua recommends with her Rejuvenating Clay to relieve lumps, cysts and tumors...Two months later on a second Mammogram, the cysts had DISAPPEARED!

Sincerely, Augusta Terzol

I went to an event at Heal Thyself Center...did not know what to expect...my life was transformed, forever. Queen educated me to cleanse...and reminded me that I am in institution in myself. She taught me that my kitchen was my laboratory; my bathroom was my spa...Queen, may you continue to be blessed with many, many more books, students and Health Centers to remake the world.

...the testimonies in your books motivate and encourage me and my friends to have an open mind... not be afraid to share our experiences... in order to overcome the many obstacles...I have learned how to heal my womb. I am no longer bitter or revengeful...learned in order to cleanse my outside appearance I must first start within.

Hotep and many blessing onto you, Michelle

I have participated in many programs with Queen Afua including the 21-Day Fast. I felt so good that I kept it up for 40 days. Queen Afua has shown great love, dedication, care, and integrity for decades; educating the community on matters of health; offering services and products of the highest quality.

~ Jean Brown, Ph.D.

Queen Afua's books never cease to bring, updated information regarding holistic healing...learned how to reduce the fibroids that plagued my entire adult life ...fasts opened my mind and expanded my awareness. I now detox on a regular basis...best part is that I learned to how to manage my emotional issues and have eliminated many of the insecurities...

...As a child I was wounded by a "loved one"... from teen to adulthood I continuously suffered from low self esteem...it seemed like the world was against me...I now know that if I want change in my life, I must change...within. I no longer carry around pains in my heart for anyone living nor deceased...making a conscious effort to forgive them truly helped me make a clean start...I can conquer any challenge that life has to offer...each day is beginning anew and brings cause for celebration. Now I am able to do lift my glass of green juice and toast to my healthy outlook on this gift called life.

...I already considered myself a healthy person, but the cleanse method Queen Afua s teaches propelled me to deepen my understanding of health and consciousness. I lost excess weight...my skin glowed...achieved great levels of inner peace and forgiveness with myself and those who have caused me pain... Much love and gratitude, Marian Isel Barragán Holistic Health Counselor I absolutely love Queen Afua and ...eloquently written words, recipes...for wellness. Thank you for being bold enough to share the truth that will continue to free so many others who are on the path to purity and purpose.

Love, Kyra Williams (Herbalist-In-Training Sacred Dancer, Educator, Mom)

I have been so enlightened by Queen's teachings. This has caused me to take a look myself...realistically. Stop all the lying and hating myself. I embrace and am learning to cherish EVERYTHING that makes me unique.

It does my soul good to know that you are teaching people how to love and heal themselves... One Truth ~ Many Paths.

Peace~Health~Contentment, Anita Foster Lovely

Queen Afua, you have...transformed my life. Your teachings are life-fulfilling skills and techniques that enable one to obtain their best possible self...they are universal and speak to the heart, soul, mind and spirit of every man, woman, boy and girl.

Blessings & Peace Minister Duroseau

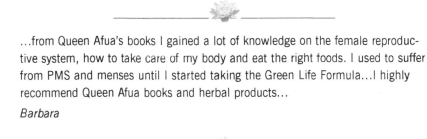

...from Queen Afua's books I gained a lot of knowledge on the female reproductive system, how to take care of my body and eat the right foods. I used to suffer from PMS and menses until I started taking the Green Life Formula...I highly recommend Queen Afua books and herbal products...

Barbara

...Queen Afua's teaching... that anyone can use it regardless of race, religion or nationality and expect to see desirable results. I think it is very fitting that she is embarking on her world tour to create a world of wellness with her universal teachings.

Sincerely, Barbara Sheri McCray

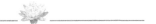

... I wrote a letter to my womb for forgiveness....Thank you, Queen Afua, for blessing us with "pure" wisdom.

Chalise Simmons San Diego CA

I was a Chemistry Major at UCLA when I heard an interview of Queen Afua on the radio... hearing this was a turning point in my life...I read her teachings of affirmations, prayer, fasting, and natural living to help purify. Truly, liberation is achieved through purification. My health is better, my self esteem is better, opportunities abound around me... I have left the field of Chemistry. ... I was given the opportunity to go to New York and visit Queen Afua's Wellness Institute. (I WAS THE WHITE GIRL!). When I walked into the center I cried. Queen Afua is my hero. I am so grateful that she has taught me so much, and that God was able to get my attention through her.

Love, Shea Stella

...I know that raw, fresh plant foods, clean water, clean air and sunlight are the keys to physical, mental and spiritual renewal...but the essential is going within to listen to your body, observe your thoughts and cultivate your spirit. A clean and vitalized body is necessary.

Thank you, Akosua Albritton

...It was because of Queen Afua's example that I founded House of Transformation in Memphis. I always ...give her credit for helping me to find the powerful feminine energy that I was able to tap into to become the woman I am today.

PEACE/LIGHT/LOVE. Sadio Bomani/ Memphis, TN

Dear Queen Afua,

I have held onto Heal Thyself...as a reference...bible for over eight years until the edges of my book are frayed...I have copied text for my mother, other women, even male friends on how to get rid of fibroids, tumors, cleanse or just make healthy drinks. I thank you from the bottom of my heart for doing the type of work that you do and for sharing your journey with us along the way.

Many Blessings! Nioka Workman

Greetings Queen Afua,

My testimony... I was told there was a lump in my breast. They drew on my breast with a red marker. They wanted to cut and take a sample to see if it was cancerous. I was so upset; I refused to let them sample any of my tissue. Instead I went to a bookstore and purchased your book, Sacred Woman. I begin to slowly go through the text. ...I rubbed my breast in red clay and almond oil and made changes in my diet. Months later I went for a mammogram and the lump was gone. No trace at all! I also made changes in how I felt about myself, body & soul. I have The "Most High" and you to thank for that.

Peace & Blessings, Annette Diop

THE MEN SPEAK

Hotep,

I want to express my love and gratitude for Queen Afua. Queen Afua has been such a blessing to my family and me for several years. During one of the roughest times of my life, as a single father, my youngest daughter contracted HIV. With the help of Queen Afua's spiritual counseling and natural herbal formulas, I'm proud to say, 7 years later, that my daughter still has no trace of HIV in her body! It only took 30 days to rid my daughter from the virus back in 2003! At that point, I knew that the creator had brought Queen Afua into my life for a divine purpose. Queen is one of the reasons I became a Certified Holistic Health Counselor and am now studying to become a Holistic Health Nutritionist. My ultimate goal is to become a Naturopath Doctor. I truly thank Queen Afua for the inspiration and personal assistance she has given me over the years!

Sincerely,
Hru Unikh Imhotep Atn Ra C.H.H.C, Divine Sacred Kingman

"Even a smile to a brother can make you feel better. The *sistahs* are scaring the men away. Even the way a *sistah* would look at you as she's walking on the street she gives you a look full of anger. 65% of Black men in the UK date outside of their race; that's something we have to pay attention to. What's the message?

The *sistas* are independent, they have all the material things they need; but they are angry...all they show is anger."

Tony Fairweather/Fairweather Productions UK
(Producer of: In Celebration of My Sisters)

From Entrfied (30 plus-year-old musician/"Baby's Daddy"):

"I am a man and have an angry vagina...she is my baby's mama, my mother, my ex-mate, my current mate ...

If I do everything in my power to do right by my daughter hopefully, she will not inherit an angry vagina..."

In the woman you have the true church of God! Why, because there is no other temple that man can enter and come out with new life. If her mate enters her mind with the true love and light of God, then all that she creates will reflect that immaculate concept.

Unfortunately, men, as whole, have become morally impotent. When a man puts no worthy spiritual cultivation in the soil of the woman, he receives no worthy harvest; nothing that will insure his divine immortality.

Immortality is not merely the continued existence of the spirit, but of one's identity throughout incarnations. A woman's gift to true love is immortality! All the problems that exist in the world can be solved at the blink of her eye, but only when the man serves the woman God from his menu (mind).

Hotep from TaharQa and Tunde Ra Aleem

How to Form Womb Wellness Circles

$\mathcal{N}$ow that you have read the stories consider creating and/or joining a womb wellness circle.

Who should form Womb Wellness Circles?
Whether a woman has a stressed out womb *or* a happy womb; has been beaten down *or* has been lifted up,

a Womb Wellness Circle is for her. Women suffering with fibroid tumors or who have had a hysterectomy,

a Womb Wellness Circle is for you. Sisters, mothers, daughters, from the four directions of the globe should form Womb Wellness Circles in order to heal yourselves and your relations.

Who is a Womb Circle Gatherer?
A Womb Circle Gatherer has a big heart and a willing spirit. She brings women together to heal themselves. She creates a safe haven of confidentiality where heart and soul sharing is encouraged and supported. She understands the relationship between an angry vagina and the wellness of the womb of the mind, heart and body. Inspired from within she is a self-appointed volunteer. She may be you.

How do we set the tone for a Womb Wellness Circle Gathering?
A circle symbolizes opening the heart to heal – to forgive – to love again. A circle of women locate a space in someone's home or in a community center. Purify the space with natural cleansers and smudge with sage or frankincense & myrrh. Arrange seating (chairs or beautiful pillows) in a circle. Set a candle and a cloth as a meditation focal point. Color suggestions for the cloth and the candle: white, blue, lavender or pink.

White – purification & cleansing; blue – peace & serenity, pink – love & forgiveness and lavender –elevation of the mind and the spirit of the spirit. Light the candle.

What is the Circle Ceremony?
After lighting the candle, read the Womb Awakening Affirmation (See Epigraph) to help to begin overcoming womb issues. Visualize for a few moments the lotus seed that will grow from you as you water it with life affirming womb wellness actions. See yourself birthing yourself out of the mud; away from pain and anger, into a healthy womb of peace and balance. Place your palms over your "first eye" in the center of your forehead and recite "I bless the womb of my mind; what I

think, I create." Breathe in and out, deeply. Next, place palms over your heart and recite "I bless the womb of my heart; what I feel, I create". Breathe in and out, deeply. Now, place palms over your reproductive womb center and recite "I bless the womb of my reproductive center; what I think and feel I birth in my womb center." Again, breathe deeply. Give thanks for the unification of the wombs of your mind, your heart and your reproductive center.

How do I connect to my Inner Voice of the Womb?

From your centered place, ask the Voice of the Womb to speak to you as she gives you the formula for your womb wellness. Deeply breathe 28 rapid fire breaths for alignment. Close your eyes and go within; trust your intuition as your womb speaks through you. Communicate with your inner voice. Upon receiving your inner messages for healing write in your journals. Share your journal entries within the Womb Wellness Circle.

How do we share our Womb Stories?

Trust yourself to share your story. Open up, breathe deeply. Healing visions will unfold. Heal your heart; release the burdens, flush out the pain. Sisters, as you cry a river of tears you are healing. Rock your body to balance. Shout gratitude for overcoming. Nurture your soul to wellness. Sisters' stories will heal sisters. Write in your journals again. You are on the threshold of a new beginning.

How do we close our circle gathering?

Embrace your sisters in gratitude. Drink Women's Life Herbal Formula or a soothing herbal tea. Enjoy the tea as it quiets your soul. End the gathering by reciting a meditation. Before separating the group should schedule their next meeting place and date. Suggested times: during the new moon (new beginning); during the full moon (rebirthing); once every 28 days. For deep womb wellness work it is recommended that the circle gathers weekly over a season.

What tools should I gather for my Womb Wellness Self Care?

Perform your womb work throughout a season (84 days). Support your womb work by joining a Womb Wellness Circle and purchasing and using womb wellness products: 21 Day Detox Kit and other appropriate tools for womb wellness).

What is my Womb Wellness homework?

Eat holistically. Journal daily. Bathe and self massage 3X a week. Love yourself unconditionally. Birth your purpose. Perform Womb Yoga and Dance of the Womb Movements every sunrise and sunset. Encourage and witness and inner and outer transformation, until we meet again.

PORTAL
Three

STORM
BEFORE THE
CALM

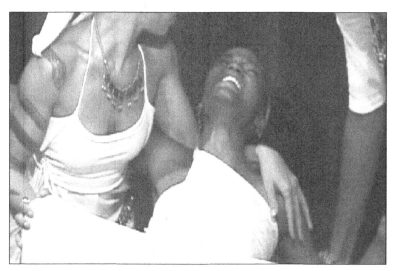

The Center of the Universe

A scene from: *The Womb Story*

CENTER OF THE UNIVERSE

The womb is the center of the universe. On the micro-level a woman's entire anatomy is connected to her womb center. On a macro-level a woman's entire life is connected to her womb center. All humans come through the womb and when our life has reached its cycle of completion on the earth plane, we transform and return into the womb of the earth. The condition of the womb is a reflection of the woman, the state of the humanity and the state of the world.

Wombs are reflections of what is about to happen and what has happened. How women are treated by a husband, life partner, mate, community and/or nation reveals levels and degrees of the "vibration" of that entity or society. When the women of a society are honored, protected and nurtured, the people, the society and the land flourish and prosper. Women who are respected, honored and loved are capable of giving birth to health, wellness, tranquility, harmony and peace. When women are *not* protected, nurtured and cared for, the land they occupy becomes barren and the people are doomed for destruction. Women treated with disdain are only capable of birthing pain and suffering, resulting in a violent, disease infested society.

Globally, there is overwhelming evidence that women have been, and continue to be abused, abandoned, bought and sold, disrespected, marginalized, mortified, mutilated, poisoned, prostituted, raped, tortured and wounded. A full study of any of these atrocities against wombs would fill many volumes and require many, many hours of discussion. Therefore, only highlights have been presented here in Portal III. Note how women are treated as property in a variety of ways in a variety of cultures. Also, note the universal similarity between acts of womb damage and existence of dis-eased wombs.

Begin to understand the correlation between global womb damage and GLOBAL ANGRY VAGINAS. Keep in mind that the compromised well-being of women announces the threat to the wellness of the global family; woman, men and children. The **selected events** in this portal is presented *for your information* as an historical timeline of circumstances that have had significant impact on women in both Western and Eastern cultures. Readers, while seeking to heal yourselves continue to research this information and the related topics. Learning the origins and impact of global interactions with women's bodies will provide a clearer understanding of the impact on women's minds, hearts, spirits and experiences. With a clearer understanding of what needs to be healed on the individual and global levels we can begin to be empowered.

IN THE BEGINNING...

Cursed: Creeds and Commandments

Cursed. Our inheritance for illness comes from a time when the balance of equality between women and men was disrupted. According to the early texts of some religions the Original Parents committed the Original Sin and were banished from the Garden of Paradise. when a woman disobeyed God's command to not eat of the fruit of knowledge, God cursed all of humanity. Because a woman had initiated the act, women were cursed to suffer great pain during menstruation and childbirth. Menstruation is even called "the curse." Doctrines based on these events developed into **creeds.**

Commandments were designed to protect society from following any of women's ideas or thoughts. Women became less than second-class citizens. Customs and taboos that followed further suppressed women's rights to define or defend themselves. In thought and in reality women were placed on pedestals and/or tied to men's rules. They became men's property and prizes. Religious creeds and social customs were codified into the laws of the state. These laws seemed as hard to break or change as the stones on which they were written. The unbalancing began.

LOCKED
Chastity and Celibacy

Chastity concerns purity of the mind and body. Traditional societies enforced chastity with commandments and customs and strong law. Young people were expected to be virgins until marriage. Married couples were expected to remain faithful to marital vows. Extra-marital sex was considered sinful, because it spiritually damaged individuals and destroyed families.

Celibacy is abstaining from all sexual activity. Laws regarding chastity and celibacy are still imposed on the faithful of all global religions, including Christianity, Islam, Buddhism, Hinduism and Confucianism. However, since the sexual revolution of the 1960s, modern Western practices have overtaken archaic mores. Today, there is widespread acceptance of unmarried sex, casual sex, "living together" instead of marriage and even extra-marital sex.

The concepts regarding chastity, abstinence and virginity is constantly evolving. However, globally women are still expected to be "pure" until marriage. Despite all modern changes in Western cultures the role-model of the bride in "virginal" white is still popular.

Chastity Belts

There are many myths about the invention and use of **chastity belts.**

What is known to be true is that they were once widely used to prevent sexual activity and even masturbation from taking place. During the 1600s, part of the European Middle Ages, husbands frequently traveled away for exploration and exploitation in foreign lands. Wives were left at home for long periods of time. It was customary for a husband to "lock down" his property – which included his home, stables, and even his wife and children. Women's wombs (wives and daughters) were "locked down" under chastity belts. It was believed that the vaginal-entrapping devices were made of iron and the key was carried away by the men. The chastity belts were not even removed during urinary evacuations and menstrual cycles. If extremely heavy iron devices and locks had been used, the lack of oxygen to the vaginal region certainly would have caused the wearers devastating infection and dis-ease and probably even death. The likelihood of chastity belts causing such severe womb damage suggests that the purpose of the chastity belt was more about the protection of men's "property" and less about the protection of women's safety and health.

Recent findings reveal that chastity belts and locks made of iron only existed in medieval poetry. By word of mouth the iron belts crossed the line from songs and tales into history books. During the Middle Ages and the Crusades the actual items used for chastity were cloth bindings and verbal or written promises. Further research reveals that the chastity belts seen in museums were produced in the early part of the 19th century as replicas of the ones described in litera-ture. Variations of the chastity belt were made in 19th century England when women purchased and used them to protect themselves from sexual harassment in the workplace.

Myth
- Women wore chastity belts made of iron and locked with a key carried away by the men.

Reality
- Chastity belts used during the time of the Crusades were cloth bindings and verbal or written promises. The earliest actual use of a leather and metal chastity garments was probably 1600s in Italy not in the 1300s.

- Iron chastity belts seen in museums in the 19th century are representa-tions of those described in literature from the earlier centuries.

- Women in 19th century England wore chastity belts to protect them-selves from sexualharassment in the workplace.

Pre-Chastity Belt. Prior to the invention of the chastity belt, there were surgical procedures used to prevent or control sexual stimulation. Infibulations, performed on women, involved sewing together of the labia majora, leaving only a small hole for urination and the passing of menstrual blood. This very small opening prevented penetration by intercourse or masturbation. Infibulations frequently caused infection, dis-ease and even death. It is arguable whether clitoridectomy practices influenced the pre-chastity belt infibulations, or if the reverse influence is the fact. Either way, again, toxic thoughts produced toxic deeds and toxic wombs. (See Female Circumcision & Genital Castration.)

Men. A little known fact is that men underwent a similar procedure, which involved the sewing together of the tip of the foreskin around the glans; also leav-ing a small hole for urination.

CINCHED

Corsets and Waist Binding

The word **corset** comes from Old French and Latin words for "body". A significant symbol of the Victorian era (1837-1901), corsets bound and shaped women's bodies and their lives. The stiff garments, worn tightly laced under close-fitting clothing, represented the stiff standards of the "upper class". A woman who wore corsets was considered a *lady* of "correct stature" and "high society" who had/would have a wealthy husband. She did not do housework or child-care. Even pregnant women wore abdominal corsets to maintain a "bound", contained look.

Fleshy body bulges were unacceptable and associated with the servants and lower classes. In the Victorian era even children wore children's corsets to prepare them for the same class of their parents. Victorian era class women were not allowed to vote and had no say about their sexuality.

Victorian Age morality descended from the mind-set of the chastity-belt era. Women were property. Sexual pleasure was for men to enjoy and women to provide. Fashion of the day demanded women's legs to be completely covered. a glimpse of a lady's ankles caused a man delight. Seeing a woman in a corset was an extra "treat". From those days to these, descendents of the corset include long-line brassieres and bustiers.

Contemporary times. Although in contemporary times wearing a waist-cinching garment generally is a woman's choice, remnants of the original patriarchal domination and class elitisms of the Victorian Age remain. Long-line brassieres, bustiers, girdles and other body shapers still are designed to hide bulges which are still symbols of the "low-class" and less sophisticated. Also note that the purpose of binding undergarments still is to "contain" the wearer, regardless of her class.

Women, be mindful that the wearing of excessively tight corsets can cause womb blockage resulting from circulatory impairment. This can manifest as increased menstrual cramps, womb numbing, and womb congestion and can even contribute to the inability to conceive due to circulatory impairment.

Related item to consider: Consistent wearing of **stiletto high-heeled shoes** can cause compromised ability to walk, compromised posture and compromised skeletal strain. Over time, the wearing of these shoes can contribute to a prolapsed or tilted womb that in chronic cases can lead to hysterectomy.

BOUND

Foot Binding

Foot binding of women and girls began in China around the 10th century and lasted for nearly one thousand years to the beginning of the 20th century. The process of foot binding, which stopped the growth of the feet, began as a luxury among the rich and soon became a prerequisite for marriage. It made women more dependant on others and less useful around the house. Binding was usually done to girls between the ages of four and seven. If the family was poor and needed their daughter's help around the house or farm, binding was done when she was older. The bandages were wrapped and tightened each day. The girl was made to wear smaller and smaller sized shoes. Bound feet had to be bathed, manicured and massaged to prevent poor circulation, gangrene and blood poisoning. After two-years the feet were very small and useless.

The erotic effect of a women's tiny bound foot has been compared to the erotic effect of a firm bosom. Also, the way foot binding made a woman walk strengthened her vaginal muscles. It is said that her "jade gate" developed to the point that she could grip her husband's "jade spear" more tightly. Erotic writings from this period express an obsession for small feet. In yet another culture we see the links among class, privilege and women as property.

Voices Against Foot Binding: In 1895, the first anti-foot binding society was formed in Shanghai. Soon, branches of the anti-foot binding society began to form in major cities throughout China.

TAKEN

Rape and Racism Related to Enslavement

Chattel enslavement was the Trans-Atlantic Slave Trade the 1400s to 1800s. It was a kind of slavery the world had not seen before. Kidnapped Africans were stripped of their humanity; not allowed to use their family-given names, speak their languages or pray to their gods. Children were separated from their families. Women were sexually abused.

Transported on ships from Africa to the Western Hemisphere, the enslaved were packed together like sardines in a can. They could not stand or walk around. Bound together they often had to lie in each other's feces, urine, and even blood. Healthy men, women and children were suddenly trapped in onboard breeding grounds for disease. Slave traders did not want disease to kill off the "cargo" and therefore, the dead and dying were thrown overboard. The Atlantic Ocean became a watery grave for thousands of Africans on the way to America through the "Middle Passage". They must have been terrified...and angry.

On the plantations stolen Africans were beaten to provide free labor from sun up to sun down in the heat of summer and the freezing winter. They were merciless-ly whipped and/or mutilated for trying to escape. The captors were sexual preda-tors feeding on African women (and men) for their own perverted pleasure. Enslaved African men were forced to be **studs** and impregnate enslaved African women. It did not matter if the women were their mothers, aunts or even their daughters. Whether the father was "master" or "slave", the babies were born into enslavement. These practices ensured a constant population of free workers. **Institutionalized racism** occurred when laws were written which allowed sexual abuses and other forms of dehumanization.

Physically, emotionally and psychologically, kidnapped African people (and their descendants) throughout the Diaspora have been damaged. As well, those who enslaved and *their* descendants have been damaged. The horrible legacy became men, controlling "their women" through sexual brutality and dysfunction. In too many families male relatives committed acts of sexual abuse in back rooms, in front rooms....sometimes even in the dark corners of the church yard. Rapes were committed while nothing was said or done to stop the brutality and the incestuous cycle. Human rights were violated. Bodies, minds and souls were vio-lated. Dis-eases were created.

Currently, diabolical and destructive behavior is the reflection and the accumulation of several generations of pre and post enslavement. It is appropriate to also remember and compare the diabolical genocidal behavior against the Indigenous populations (Native Americans) in the Western Hemisphere.

There are obvious correlations between the subhuman treatments experienced by enslaved Africans, especially the horror of being forced to rape one's own daughter, sister or mother and the multiple dysfunctions in African American families in particular and American families in general. Four hundred years of chattel enslavement, followed by plantation captivity and institutionalized racism have been major factors in the making of damaged wombs and angry vaginas in the United States. These human disgraces leave a stain on everybody's hands and damage in all wombs.

CUT
Female Genital Cutting (FGC)

The origins of **female genital cutting (FGC)** are somewhat of a mystery. The practice transcends religion, geography, and socio-economic status. It is believed to have existed in parts of ancient Africa, Asia (in countries now known as the Middle East) and European countries.

FGC is performed on girls usually between the age the ages of 6 and 12 years. Midwives or those trained to perform circumcisions go from village to village and perform the cutting without anesthesia or antibiotics. Unsterilized instruments for cutting and burning are reused from patient to patient. After the tissue is cut, salves made of ingredients such as honey or tree sap are used on open wounds to ease the bleeding. The most common immediate complication is uncontrolled bleeding. Complications include fever and infections due to unsterilized tools and conditions. Girls who have undergone Type I usually heal within a few days. Girls who have undergone Type III require bed rest for about one week. Their thighs and legs are bound together to ensure proper *healing* of the infibulated scar. The most common long-term complications are recurrent vaginal and urinary tract infections, infertility, cysts, abscesses, keloid formation, difficult labor and delivery, and sexual dysfunction. Many women and girls have died during soon after FGC procedures.

According to WHO (World Health Organization) there are four types of FGC:
Type I: Clitoridectomy or sunna – removal of part or all of the clitoris.

Type II: Excision, involves removing part or all of the clitoris and labia minora.

Type III: Infibulation or pharaonic – the most severe form – removal of part or all of the external genitalia and narrowing the vaginal orifice. The infibulated scar covers the urethra and leaves only a small hole for urination and menses.

Type IV: Any harm done to the genitalia by pricking, piercing, cutting, scraping, or burning. This is the physically least invasive form.

Women with Type III FGC can be offered a defibulation procedure. Defibulation, a surgical procedure performed under regional or general anesthesia, reopens the infibulated scar.

As late as the 1960s, American obstetricians performed clitoridectomies to "treat" lesbianism, hysteria, and clitoral enlargement. More than 130 million women worldwide have undergone FGC. FGC occurs in parts of Africa and Asia, in societies with various cultures and religions. Reasons for the continuing practice of FGC include rite of passage, preserving chastity, ensuring marriage-ability, religious mandates, hygiene, improving fertility and enhancing sexual pleasure for men. Yet, again the woman's womb is for men's pleasure and ownership. The circumstances for the creation of angry vaginas are astounding and exist in the millions.

Female Circumcision & Genital Castration—Realties & Facts

- Annually 2,000,000+ women are circumcised; every 16 seconds a female child is circumscribed. Worldwide 100 million females have been genitally mutilated.

- As a result of immigration, FGC has also spread to Europe, Australia and the US. Some families have their daughters undergo FGM during visits to their home countries. As **Western governments** become more aware of FGM, they are passing legislation to make the practice of FGM a criminal offense in their country.

Voices Against Female Castration: In July, 2003 at its second summit, the African Union adopted the Maputo Protocol promoting women's rights including an end to female genital mutilation.

INSIDE
STDs and AIDS

STDs. A sexually transmitted disease (STD), sexually transmitted infection (STI) or venereal disease (VD) is an illness that is most probably transmitted between humans by means of vaginal, oral, and/or anal sexual behavior. Some STDs can also be transmitted through the use of IV (Intravenous) drug needles after they are used by an infected person. Even childbirth or breastfeeding can transmit infections from the mother to the child.

HIV and AIDS. Acquired immune deficiency syndrome (AIDS) is a disease that progressively reduces the immune system's ability to function effectively. Individuals with HIV (Human immunodeficiency virus) and AIDS can become more susceptible to opportunistic infections and tumors. HIV is transmitted through **direct contact** with bodily fluids containing HIV during vaginal, oral or anal sex, blood transfusion, shared, contaminated hypodermic needles or mother/baby exchange during pregnancy, childbirth and/or breastfeeding.

Globally, AIDS is pandemic. In 2007, it was estimated that globally, 33.2 million people lived with the disease and that AIDS killed an about 2.1 million people, including 330,000 children.

STDs and AIDS and HIV Realties & Facts
- Worldwide, 11 of every 1,000 adults between the ages 15 to 49 are HIV-infected

- In the US, among new HIV infections, approximately 75% of the women are infected through heterosexual sex, and 25% through drug related uses. Of the newly infected women—64% are of African ascent; 18% are of Indigenous/Hispanic heritage; and the remaining percentages are from other racial/ethnic groups.

- Infection rates vary enormously between countries in the same region and between urban and rural populations. In general, the prevalence of STDs tends to be higher in urban residents, in unmarried individuals, and in young adults.

Fibroid Tumors

Fibroid tumors are benign growths found on the walls of the uterus. Also called myoma, fibroid tumors may be silently present and cause no problems. However, in some women, fibroids can cause frequent menstrual periods with heavy bleeding, pelvic pain, infertility, and recurrent pregnancy loss. Severe anemia can 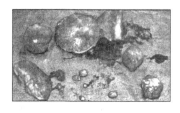 result from excessive uterine bleeding. Other symptoms can include pelvic pressure on the woman's bladder or rectum which may result in frequent urination or constipation. Some women experience pain during sexual intercourse (due to an enlarged uterus.)

Cysts and tumors

Endometriosis – a disorder of the female reproductive system in which the endometrium, which normally lines the uterus, grows in other places such as on the fallopian tubes, ovaries or the tissue lining the pelvis.

Endometrioid cyst – caused by endometriosis is a common cause of female infertility.

Hemorrhagic cyst – occurs when bleeding is present with the cyst.

Dermoid cyst – comprised of the same tissue as skin, fat, bone, hair, cartilage and even teeth; may become inflamed or cause ovarian torsion (twisting).

Polycystic ovary – usually twice its normal size with many small cysts on the outside

Fibroid tumor facts and realities:

- **In the United States:** Approximately 20-40% of women 35 years and older have fibroid tumors. Currently approximately 10-21 million women in the US have fibroids. Fibroids are more common among women of **African-American** descent. Some statistics indicate that up to 80% of African-American women will develop uterine fibroids.

- **Hispanic** women living in the US have twice the incidence rate of and 1.4 times the mortality rate from cervical cancer compared with non-Hispanic whites.

- **In the United Kingdom:** Fibroids are present in 1/4 to 1/5 of Caucasian women and 1/2 of Black women in the UK.

- **In Canada:** An Ontario Uterine Fibroid Embolization study, published in 2003 was comprised of 550 women with an average age of 43 who experienced fibroid related symptoms for more than 5 years. Many of those women were opposed to surgery and actively sought alternatives. Symptoms suffered by patients with fibroids have a great negative impact on their quality of life. Fibroids are also much more common among African-Canadian women than in Canadian women who are not of African ancestry.

REMOVED
Hysterectomies

Hysterectomy is the surgical removal of the uterus due to enlarged tumors, and chronic womb bleeding primarily caused by fibroid tumors. Fibroid tumors are the leading cause of hysterectomies being performed. Women are receiving hysterectomies at increasing alarming rates. The age of women receiving hysterectomies is steadily becoming younger and younger. About 25% of women aged 25-50 years have fibroids. The number doubles to 50% in the African-American community. According to the US National Uterine Fibroids Foundation, every ten minutes twelve hysterectomies are performed. In addition to the health concerns there is also a large economic factor associated with this surgical procedure. Annually about 5 billion dollars is spent in medical expenses on hysterectomies. Personally, since it takes women about six weeks to recover, each woman loses about 1,200 hours of work. Risk factors can also be high with approximately 660 women dying each year in the due to complications from a hysterectomy.

Hysterectomy Realities & Facts
- **In the United States** – Annually 600,000+ women have hysterectomies

- **In the United States** – In the last 20 years, over 12 million have had hysterectomies

- **In the United States** – Every 10 minutes there are 12 hysterectomies performed

- **Globally** – Annually 2,000,000+ women have legal and illegal hysterectomies performed

- **Globally** – Annually as many as 366,000 fibroid cases end with hysterectomies

- **Globally** – for every 10,000 hysterectomies performed, 11 women die.

CHANGED

Menopause

Menopause is the part of a woman's life when the menstrual periods permanently end. This happens because as a woman ages, her ovaries make less of the female hormones estrogen and progesterone. Menopause is a major health issue that has become an unnatural dis-ease due to the lack of proper health care and resources for most women in both "developed" and "underdeveloped" countries, globally. More than 70% of the world's population of women who experience menopause do not have, do not know and/ or do not use treatments to address the hormonal imbalances. Conditions associated with menopause are many and varied. Not all women get all or any of the symptoms.

Symptoms usually associated with menopause include:
- Periods become longer or shorter or heavier or lighter or missed periods
- Hot flashes
- Palpitations
- Night sweats
- Vaginal dryness

- Dry skin
- Insomnia and other sleep disturbances,
- Mood swings; Crying for no apparent reason; General irritability and/or anger
- Depression
- Anxiety and/or Panic attacks
- Hair thinning or loss
- Pain during sex
- Frequent urinary infections; Urinary incontinence
- Decreased or non-existent libido
- Increase in body fat especially around the waist
- Problems with concentration and memory

Menopause Realities & Facts

- **In the US** an estimated 35.2 million women experienced menopause in 2003 in comparison to the 28.7 million who experienced it in 1990. It has been estimated that by 2020 more than 45 million women will have experienced menopause and accept as "normal" the imbalances and dis-eases associated with menopause.

- In the US, 75% plus of menopausal women are experiencing more severe hormonal imbalances despite using synthetic pharmaceutical drugs to "balance" their physiological womb issues.

- **Globally:** There are insufficient studies being done regarding the pre and post menopausal realties of women. This is particularly true in underdeveloped nations.

MORE CAUSES OF ANGRY VAGINAS

- C.R.A.C.K. is a program that pays addicted women $200 to be sterilized
  http://cwpe.org/files/crackingcrack-scully.pdf.

- The Puerto Rican Sterilization Project discusses the violations against the Puerto Rican women's rights for reproductive freedom and matters of fertility.
  http://muse.jhu.edu/login?uri=/journals/nwsa_journal/v021/21.3.martinez.html

- Forced sterilization laws in the early 1900s in the US

- Forced Sterilizations of Native American woman in 60s and 70s.

- Forced sterilization and forced abortions of women in prison in the US
  http://www.facinghistory.org/resources/rm

- Birth control methods –devices, injections and oral contraceptive pre-scriptions that cause unnatural and harmful incidences in the body

These are circumstances of women's lack of control over their own bodies. They are conditions of imbalance that render women susceptible to developing womb damage and angry vaginas.

...AND STILL MORE CAUSES OF ANGRY VAGINAS

- Sexual Abuse and Rape not related to enslavement
- Incest not related to enslavement
- Fairy Tale Complex: When women seek to emulate Sleeping Beauty, Cinderella, Snow White. roles taught in childhood in the hope of becoming beautiful, un-resourceful maidens who get rescued by handsome, ever-resourceful princes.
- Disenfranchisement (Joblessness, Homelessness, Poverty)
- Single motherhood
- Incarceration
- Obesity and related symptoms
- Anorexia and related symptoms
- Image: Self-Esteem vs. Social Demands
- Depression and Mental Illnesses
- Substance Abuse
- Cancer
- Suicide

Volumes have been written about these and related causes of angry vaginas. As said about the topics presented above, these are circumstances where imbalance is present and empowerment is severely challenged or altogether absent.

WOMB JOURNEY TIMELINE

Below is a time line of storms and *dis*-eases that *could* challenge the journey of a woman's womb life. When unaware of these pitfalls, a woman is less able to protect, much less heal herself. Even if she *is* aware she may remain "stuck in the mud" until her awareness guides her to heal herself and/or to inform and protect others. By embracing the strategies suggested in the five portals of this text one may be able to avoid or convert the traumas of a negative womb journey into the liberation of the positive journey of conscious womb-wellness.

The beginning/Pre-birth Negative issues passed sperm to ovum through the bloodline	**7 – 16 years old** Incest	**14 years old** Traumatic teenage sexual encounter with toxic, confused partner
16 years old STDs	**16 – 30 years old** Infertility; Miscarriages; Abortion as a form of birth control	**13 – 40 years old** PMS; Heavy menstrual bleeding, clotting, cramping; Vaginal sores, itching, burning, odor, discharge; Endometriosis
19 years old Abnormal Pap smear	**24 – 40 years old** Infertility; Difficult childbirths Miscarriages; Abortion as a form of birth control	**24 years old** Womb cysts
28 years old Fibroid tumors	**29 years old** Tumor removal (surgical or radiation)	**31 years old** Tumors grow back within 1-3 years
40 years old Prolapsed womb; Painful intercourse; Uterine cancer	**45 – 60 years old** Difficult menopause; Hot flashes; Vaginal dryness	**45 – 60+ years old** Hysterectomy

FORGIVENESS

You have traveled through three portals of overcoming an angry vagina. Diligently you seek to apply the guidance to womb wellness suggested in PORTAL ONE and to share your womb stories as inspired by those told in PORTAL TWO. The storms before the calm in PORTAL THREE were present- ed to help you better understand the challenges (mud) you might face as you prepare to overcome and bloom forth into your wellness. Now, in order to heal ourselves; to restore ourselves to wholeness and peace, we must forgive.

Woman, I invite you to break the deadly cycle of an Angry Vagina.
Man, I invite you to break the deadly cycle of a Hostile Penis.
I know that each of you are you are hurt.
I know each of you has been hurt by the other.
I invite you to speak. Come together; face to face and heart to heart to speak
  forgiveness for your recovery.
I invite us to speak so that you may forgive and love and travel through your
  bloodline to heal the past and the future.

I forgive you for the slaps and the kicks, for the grabbing and the yanking,
    for the shaking of my soul and my body, for the historical abuse
          and the global madness that birthed sick souls.
      I forgive you for the cursing and the yelling and the screaming;
    for the hostile words spoken, for the cruel tones and the harsh looks
that ruptured my veins and traveled deep into the womb of my heart.

      Will you forgive me for shattering your regeneration centre;
            for drowning us in a river of tears and regret?
        I forgive you for not keeping your word, your promise,
      I forgive you for not staying, for letting go and for holding on
                when I should have let you go.
      I forgive you for running from one womb, woman, to another.
        I forgive you for running from one man to another
    in the hope of finding salvation, even while I was there for you.
I forgive you for abandoning me, for not being there when I reached out.
  I forgive you for not speaking to me gently, when I needed comforting.
        I forgive you for holding resentment towards me,
              when it was not me who hurt you.

I, woman, forgive you for unpacking your emotional, toxic baggage
into my vagina, while using your penis as a weapon,
causing me to bleed a river of issues.
I, man, forgive you for holding onto your pain and releasing resentment
into my reproductive center, which then went to my chest,
causing my heart to fail.
I forgive you for not knowing or understanding;
for not caring what I felt or how I felt.

I, woman, forgive you for being like my daddy or not being like my daddy.
I, man, forgive you for being like my mother, or not being like my mother.

My Angry Vagina wants to overcome the pain
that has filled my inner walls
with cysts, tumors, and clotting.
My hostile penis wants peace and love; not impotency.
Can we attract the beauty that is within me and you?
Will you forgive me whether I stay or move on;
whether I hold on or let go?
May we become wiser for the lesson we have learned?
May we hold in our hearts sweet, lasting forgiveness?

I forgive you for everything.
I need soulful liberation, freed up in the rapture of forgiveness.
I need to heal. I need my wings.
I want to soar beyond the pain.
I forgive you. Will you forgive me? I forgive you. Will you forgive me?
I forgive you. Will you? Will you forgive me?
Forgive me…forgive me…forgive me…I forgive you…

As you walk the road of forgiveness the womb of your heart is expanding with wellness. You are crossing the bridge over troubled waters. Many-deserved treasures await you for your efforts and hard work. Continue to travel into the REBIRTH of your life.

PORTAL
Four

REBIRTH

*T*o Rebirth a Woman
is to Rebirth the Earth

Your Purpose,
Your Visions, Your Work

*I*n order to rebirth yourself there must be a healing between you, your purpose, your vision and your work. Rebirth yourself and receive the treasures of wholeness, harmony and prosperity. Live your truth and become fully alive, encouraged and enlightened. Avoid a life filled with frustration and lack of fulfillment; this can lead to *dis*-ease. Reclaim your purpose as an ongoing process of acknowledgement, empowerment, sharing and growth.

When your life's **work** – regardless of how grand or humble – empowers you. Expressing your natural talents and gifts, enables you to create works that support mental and physical health. By living your "right" work you can bring forth harmony and prosperity for yourself and others.

In ancient traditions, work – usually the family business – established one's destiny. Work existed according to the needs and well-being of the family and community. Infants were named in a way that kept them mindful of their life's purpose. The elders guided the youth to be in harmony with purpose; they instilled awareness that actions have a direct impact on the family, the community, and the nation.

In contemporary times there is much less access to such guidance. Most of us have no family business to inherit. Too many of us spend our formative years searching for who we are and what we are here to do. The connection to the wisdom of the elders has been lost; there is confusion and ignorance about purpose and mission. We are told to go to school and get good grades so that we may get good jobs. After years of study we receive a degree, but may end up in a job for which we have no passion; a job that does not allow us to realize our vision.

Fortunately, you do not have to remain trapped in a soul-less, unfulfilling job. There is guidance for you. Allow yourselves to be led by spirit and those close to you who can guide you. Become inspired to recreate your world. With guidance, find your purpose. Have faith. Be creative. Everything you need to create a meaningful is within your grasp.

There are times when we may hold back for fear of the scope of our visions. They may seem too vast and grand. Move beyond your fear, embrace yourself and create a plan. Be bold in spirit. Become emancipated; do not allow your job to enslave you. When you embrace success, you will grow and your work will grow. The change in your approach to your purpose will give both you and your community fulfillment and enrichment. When you are free to live your purpose you will be in a better place to live a *dis*-ease-free existence. Tumors will dissolve and high blood pressure will lower. Gratitude and joy will take over because you dared to live, not merely exist.

BIRTHING YOUR LIFE

Did you hear?

We're about to birth a new world!

Become one with yourself and your work

Birth your vision

Get in line with the Divine

The Great Spirit will guide you to your vision

Dare to step to your natural rhythm.

Let's say that you a work 40 hours weekly, 160 hours monthly, 1,920 hours yearly, on a job that feeds depression, disappointment, racism, resentment and/or rage. If you "march to the beat of another's drum," you will be out of your own rhythm. It is likely that you have a host of blockages. Your body shows this condition as you end up carrying 15–100 pounds of excess weight caused by emotions and toxins that poison your thoughts, your feelings, and your spirit. This toxic state causes one to be susceptible to high blood pressure, premature aging, strokes, heart conditions, tumors, skin eruptions, stress and depression, just to name a few *dis*-eases.

Being a conscious woman or man, you must perform the work that is your purpose. Detox and purify your body so that you can be ready to recognize yourself and your work. As a reward for your purification efforts your mission will come through loud and clear. You can unleash and birth the gift of your "right and correct" work on the earth; work that uplifts, restores, empowers, and transforms humanity into the true nature of goodness.

The Blessings of living your "right" work
Discover your truth. It may take you a lifetime to realize your correct work – and, so be it. Pray without ceasing that you may recognize your purpose when it shows up, and pray that you have the courage to birth it and know joy.

Do not settle
Search until your true work reveals itself to you. If everyone were about their correct mission, as they should be, this world would be a place not of fear, pain, frustration and *dis*-ease, but an earth and a people of light, joy, wellness, and abundance – equally shared.

How do you know?

You know your life's work when you are in love with it. Your great love for your work will draw support and abundance. When you discover your work, you want to do it all the time. Your life's work feeds and nourishes your soul with wholeness, peace, power and yes, even with prosperity. Stay loyal to your calling even if it takes a lifetime. Accept your calling with a resolved state of courage. Go forth with your work and really begin to really live.

Ishe Oluwa Koleba Jeo

(The Most High's Work is indestructible)

An example of living your "right and correct" work from Queen Afua:
In the 1960s, I became involved in the glorious a time of revolutionaries and activists seeking truth, freedom and self-knowledge. I studied and performed African dance. My formal studies led me to become a Hatha Yoga teacher, wholistic health consultant, fasting instructor, colon therapist, polarity practitioner and lay midwife. Yes, I am a healer and an author and an artist. I have been blessed to recognize the unlimited dimensions of every possibility to birth that which is inside of me. You can as well.

On January 23rd, 2003 at Howard University in Washington D.C., I was center stage about to perform a sacred dance I had choreographed. I was doing what I loved best. The curtains came up. The lights shined down on my dance company, Abut em Khat Ankhsamble. What a wonder! We were the opening performance for the National Black Dance Conference.

We danced our visions from out of our souls. We performed the Nile Valley River Dance (early stages of the Womb Yoga Dance presented in Portal Five of this text). Some had tried to limit me with fears and doubts, "Stay in the box," they whispered. My spirit said, "Let me go free. I am here to encourage you to stand strong in your vision."

Know that you will hit rocks and bumps along the way; you will climb steep hills to reach yourself. Regardless of the obstacles, rise. Move courageously forward. What appear as obstacles are but the lessons needed to help you cultivate your vision/work.

Open up soulfully and allow the divine in you to walk you through your glorious and most fulfilling vision/work. You can make it happen, just trust. Listen from within as you allow yourself to be spiritually guided to your vision/work – your dearest friend.

BIRTHING BLUES

Blockages

Birthing Blues (blockages and crises) indicate the lack of preparation and readiness to conceive, carry and deliver your work. What is blocking you? What are your birthing blues and how can heal from them? All the answers are inside of you.

To overcome challenges keeping you from your goals become attuned to your dream and make it a reality. Answer these questions and begin form a clear picture of what is blocking your success. Learn what must be unblocked and overcome in order for you to manifest your visions.

Birthing Blues Song

Do you sometimes sing the Birthing Blues Song?

I don't have enough money

I don't have energy after work

I don't have support from my family

I am afraid to act, because I will probably fail anyway

I have a secure job with benefits, why rock the boat

I don't deserve or believe that I can do what I really want to do

I don't have a degree in the area of work that I want to do

Stop singing that song! You don't have to have *all* the resources you will need in order to begin pursuing your vision. Get started; use what you have; build your vision one brick at a time. The elders used to say; "If life gives you lemons, make lemonade." Make wonderful lemonade.

Childhood Approval Syndrome. Answer the following questions:

- In my youth, did anyone encourage or discourage me from living my life's work?

- Who and how?

- In my adulthood, who encouraged and who discouraged me?

- What are some of the hurdles that I must overcome to live my vision?

- What are my fears about living my vision, my purpose?

- How long have I been in fear about living my purpose?

Discard limitations imposed on you in your childhood. Discard phrases that block you: "Don't go outside the box..." "You can't..." Our parents/elders taught us *their* visions for us. Although we may not have always believed in their visions, they definitely had an impact on who we became. Right, or wrong, or in between, it is time to develop our own visions for ourselves. Clean up and get away from whatever has stopped you from living your divine, powerful destiny.

Beware

Watch out who you tell about your vision. It is neither wise nor necessary to "tell all" before you properly prepared. People may try to discourage you. They may not be able to see what you see. Choose friends and company carefully. Choose people who reflect your ideals and can help you to form and birth your vision.

Believe in yourself.

Clean up: These are some of the dis-eases that are signs that we are neither living our purpose nor doing our work. They form a vicious cycle cause and effect of illness.

- Drug or alcohol abuse
- Infertility
- Impotency
- Migraine headaches
- Obesity
- Ulcers
- Anxiety due to being overwhelmed
- Misplaced work/wrong choice of work
- Going from job to job
- Overworked, underpaid
- Unhappy about work environment
- Work is not economically prosperous
- Working in a dead-end job

Identifying these blockages is the beginning of conceiving and birthing your vision work.

BLOCKAGES QUESTIONNAIRE

Time: _____ Date: _____

Ask yourself the following questions:

Right now, am I satisfied and in alignment with my work and my life's mission:
❑ No   ❑ Yes

Blockages to my vision work:

Yes	No	
❑	❑	My work makes me feel ill, depressed and angry.
❑	❑	When at work, I wish I were elsewhere.
❑	❑	I am not living out my life's work/mission.
❑	❑	I keep making excuses for why I think I can't succeed.
❑	❑	I feel my mission is unable to feed, clothe, and support me.
❑	❑	I am working a dead-end job.
❑	❑	I am dissatisfied with my work.

Yes	No	
❑	❑	I dislike the people I work with.
❑	❑	I feel consistently overwhelmed in my work.
❑	❑	My current work suppresses my creativity.
❑	❑	I feel stifled in my current job.
❑	❑	I feel jealous of others.
❑	❑	I feel abusive toward others.
❑	❑	I am in mental or spiritual pain.
❑	❑	I feel confused.

Checking "Yes", to two or more of these items, indicates danger of not being ready to birth your vision work. However, you can begin to get ready.

CHALLENGES TO
YOUR BIRTHING VISION

*C*onsider the challenges that a woman may face as she prepares to conceive, carry and give birth to a child. Your purpose, your vision is your child. Examine the challenges so that you can recognize them if they appear and attempt to prevent you from birthing your purpose and vision. You can prepare yourself to overcome the challenges (mud) and bloom yourself and your work into glorious triumph (lotus blossoms). But first, let us study what we must overcome.

Infertility – is when one cannot begin to conceive a vision. Infertility is mental, physical and/or emotional stagnation. It is the feeling of not being enough, having enough or knowing enough.

Affirmation (Antidote):
Divine light dwells in me. I affirm today that I am enough, I have enough, and I know enough. I'm open enough to unblock myself and birth my vision.

Abortion – Indicates that the seed and egg of your vision was germinated. You conceived, but after conception, you felt hopelessness, fear or lack of preparation. You felt you didn't have what it takes to support your vision. You terminated your vision.

Affirmation (Antidote):
I affirm I am not longer scared of birthing my vision. I embrace myself completely; therefore I will absolutely prepare myself to carry my vision to full-term.

Miscarriage (Spontaneous abortion) – Indicates the weight of your vision was too heavy to carry. One must develop the "muscle", the conscience and skills to carry ones vision.

Affirmation (Antidote):
Because I nurtured myself appropriately I have the power to carry the weight and force of my vision work.

Morning Sickness – indicates a lack of preparation for your purpose. You experience a state of *dis*-ease due to a lack of mental, physical and spiritual cleansing before conception.

Affirmation (Antidote):
My temple is pure, healthy and united in body, mind and spirit. I am capable of preventing morning sickness.

Edema/preeclampsia – indicates being extremely overwhelmed by your vision. Absolutely challenged about carrying your work, you become poisoned by it. Your vision was conceived in fear and negativity, which continues throughout the "pregnancy" and causes the shut down of your capacity to create.

Affirmation (Antidote):
My purpose and I are in Divine Order. I have replaced the fears and doubts of carrying and birthing my purpose with confidence and strength.

Premature Birth – indicates that your underdeveloped vision was born too soon. By grace, it lives. Your vision requires extreme care in order to survive to maturity.

Affirmation (Antidote):
My vision is developed, strong and powerful. This is accomplished through absolute love, devotion, dedication and care for the coming forth of my vision.

Still-born – indicates lack of nourishment or faith, knowledge (training), and enthusiasm. You fear you are not enough to carry your vision to its zenith. You carried your vision full term, but on its birth it died due to the lack syndrome.

Affirmation (Antidote):
My vision is alive and well. I have faith, knowledge, enthusiasm and support to maintain and grow my vision.

Crib Death – the death of your vision came after birth. Now that the vision is born, you are still lacking the appropriate knowledge of your purpose and its needs, so it dies unexpectedly. Crib death of your vision indicates a lack of appropriate support, (i.e., promotion, economics, love, nurturing); your vision was short lived.

Affirmation (Antidote):
I affirm that my vision lives though me, fully alive. Daily I strengthen my vision as I grow, expand and breathe appreciation, joy and vitality into purpose.

Hysterectomy – indicates that your vision is in danger of never being born. It indicates that the opportunity for your vision has been completely rooted out, and you are now convinced that you will never manifest your vision.

Affirmation (Antidote):
My work vision is rooted firmly within me. Nothing, no one, not even I, will hinder the conception and the birth of my divine vision.

Beloved Women and Men on the quest for balance and rebirth:
Use the information in this portal to help you prevent and overcome blockages and challenges. Remember, you are a lotus seed in the mud of challenge. Create the destiny to rebirth yourself, your purpose, your vision and your work.

OVERCOMING
THE BIRTHING BLUES

*B*irthing Blues blockages prevent finding one's purpose. Birthing Blues challenges destroy visions. Birthing Blues blockages and Birthing Blues challenges are due to due to a lack of preparation. Use strategies and tools for developing and living a Natural Lifestyle in order to get ready to conceive and birth your purpose, your vision, your work.

Continue to recite daily affirmations:

- I accept that I am overcoming all birthing traumas.

- I accept that I will open myself up to healing beyond the Birthing Blues.

- I accept my purpose, my vision, my work with courage.

- I am one with my purpose.

- My vision is my service to the enhancement of humanity.

- My vision is my passion.

- I have unwavering faith that I will go full term and birth vision.

- I am entitled to and deserve to live my purpose.

- My vision and work, no matter how humble or grand, is my service to the Divine.

If you are still unclear about your work, then seek consul from someone you trust. Refer to a priest, priestess, minister, spiritualist, astrologer, numerologist, or your local "bush doctor" for guidance and direction. Remember to ask the elders to help you. Even just listening to a story they have to tell might spark something you need to hear and know. Do not be afraid to ask for help. Be confident that you have something to offer to the community once you begin your creative work. Realize that discovering your creative work, is profoundly intertwined with finding your true self and living your life correctly and fully.

All that you need to birth your vision is inside of you. Think pure thoughts, eat pure foods, and perform pure actions in order to nourish the seed of your creative work. Detox and rejuvenate through fasting. Get up early in the morning and listen deeply to your heart and mind. The answers that you seek about your purpose will be revealed to you in the detail that you need.

Positive Characteristics
for Those Who Dare to Live Their Purpose

Work on developing these characteristics within yourself. Look for these characteristics in others to help you identify those who are living their vision and dong their work.

- ❏ Excited about living
- ❏ Creative
- ❏ Enjoy good health
- ❏ Joyous
- ❏ Fulfilled
- ❏ Free
- ❏ Radiant
- ❏ Unlimited vision
- ❏ Loving
- ❏ Have sufficient income to live their vision

A Rebirthing Story

August 2007: I woke up with a shooting pain in my back and my legs that made me shriek. I could not stand. In the emergency room, I was x-rayed, and questioned, and finally given disturbing news. The doctor said that I had two herniated discs in my lumbar area and rheumatoid arthritis in my spine. He said the illnesses were hereditary and eventually I would not be able to walk.

Inside my spirit, the Creator whispered, *"The only thing that is hereditary is your lifestyle, change your lifestyle."* The doctor mentioned surgery; I opted for physical therapy. Through PT I increased my endurance, lost weight and began taking my well-being very seriously.

September 2007: I started a new job. In two months my weight increased to 240 pounds because I had to stop PT, I had additional stress and I did not know enough about healthy eating.

January 2008: My co-worker encouraged me to start a cleansing program. I struggled, but my support team stood by me. I lost 20 pounds. While detoxing my mind felt clear and light. I was euphoric. My focus had been to lose weight, be well, think well and speak well. I prayed for a path to open up and for new opportunities.

March 2008: A friend introduced me to *The City of Wellness: Restoring Your Health Through the Seven Kitchens of Consciousness* by Queen Afua. The book shifted my path forever. I discovered a new me, a whole me, a well me; I have not turned back. I applied what I learned, removed all meats from my diet. My body ached less, I was less angry, I was sleeping better and I had more energy. I received the step-by-step guide for my husband, my children and myself to live a more wholistic way.

September 2009: I decided to register for the Emerald Green Practitioner Certification with Queen Afua and made plans to pilgrimage to New York.

November 2009: I was notified that the class was canceled. It took my breath away. I called Queen Afua. After many days of meditating I decided to sponsor Queen Afua to come to Columbus, Ohio for 3 days of wellness.My goal set me on a fierce mission. A new authority, courage, faith and energy emerged from me that I had never seen before. I was breaking through blockages that kept me from achieving my greatness. I uncovered wellness for my family, my community and myself. I broke down walls, improved communication, formed wellness circles and created bonds of support and encouragement that still remain in tact.

January of 2010: I have completed 365 days of cleansing. I had shed 95 pounds. Currently, I weigh a beautiful 145 pounds and my back no longer gives me any troubles. Today, I am a walking testimony to Natural Living Lifestyle. I have taken control of my wellness. And, yes, I achieved my certification as an Emerald Green Practitioner of Wellness. I am committed to the wellness of my family, my city, my state and beyond. I give praise and thanks for the Most High blessing me with a supportive mate who is on this wellness journey with me. I rebirthed myself. All praises to the Creator and love to Queen Afua!

Respectfully, Nancy Minter "Queen Freedom", Columbus, OH

Conceive Your Vision

It is time to create an inner environment in which to nurture the seeds of your purpose and work. You are reminded to **purify** in order to conceive, maintain and birth balanced thoughts for a clear and correct vision. You are reminded to focus.

Center your creative energy.

Open yourself up to inner spiritual guidance.

Clear your energy field of negative thoughts/ emotions/ reactions/ relations.

Imagine the *conception* of your vision of your work as inspired communication between you and your understanding of your purpose. It is intercourse between light and your dreams. To best prepare for the conception cleanse, pray and trust;

open yourself up to receive the light and the dream. Do not be afraid.

If fear blocks the conception, breathe the breath of trust and acceptance. Relax and let go in order to conceive the fullness of your purpose. Affirm daily: *The energy field inside of the womb of my mind is filled with light.*

As you prepare to conceive your vision, recite affirmations in rounds alternating with deep breathing to bring air into the womb of you mind and heart.

Round I:

- I release hostility (breathe) from the womb of my mind.

- I release rage (breathe) from the womb of my mind.

- I release insecurity (breathe) from the womb of my mind.

- I release hurt (breathe) from the womb of my mind.

- I release resentment (breathe) from the womb of my mind.

- I release fear (breathe) from the womb of my mind.

- I release doubt (breathe) from the womb of my mind.

Round II.

- I bring the breath of light into the womb of my mind.

- I bring the breath of love into the womb of my mind.

- I bring the breath of serenity into the womb of my mind.

- I bring the breath of peace into the womb of my mind.

- I bring the breath of strength into the womb of my mind.

- I bring the breath of joy into the womb of my mind.

- I bring the breath of pure energy into the womb of my mind

The light of your vision will begin to swell. Continue to breathe deeper. The light of your vision will become stronger. You vision will become a fire inside of the womb of your mind. It will expand and impregnate the womb of your heart. It is there! The vision has been planted. Its potential is unlimited. You have conceived yourself. You are in the birthing house; you are with child. Become devoted to carrying your vision through all the cycles as you grow the vision inside of your-self, is protected within your body temple. Nurture your vision daily. Look forward to giving birth to a radiant beautiful, profound, crystal clear vision, Everyone will come from far and near to share in your vision.

Carrying Your Vision

You are growing. Be confident; your vision is getting stronger. Continue to act on faith, and know that all you will need to bring forth your work will be given to you as you grow into your true self, through pure natural living and being.

The gestation period for your vision could take from a minimum of 9 weeks and as long as 9 months. The number 9 represents completion, coming of age, going full circle indicating that your vision has fully ripened. Below are activities to strengthen the body mind and spirit during the gestation period.

Keep yourself encircled by people you want to emulate; who encourage and inspire you to grow

Take intensive training to support your sacred work vision. The more knowledge and skills you acquire in your field, the more confident and secure your birth.

Volunteer in the field of your calling for on-the-job hands on experience and training.

Strengthen your business plan.

Become a part of associations that focus on your career.

Embellish and perfect your plans. It may take several drafts before you reach your final document. The more clear and precise your mission statement, the better the manifestation of your work will be.

Sweat it out in a sauna or a steam bath for one hour off and on between showers as you wash your doubts away, 1–2 times a week or as often as necessary to keep yourself receptive to birthing your vision.

Keep your body well-nourished and cleansed daily.

Drink 8–12 oz. of freshly pressed fruit juices with 8–12 ounces of distilled water daily plus one quart of warm water with the juice of 2 limes or lemons. As you drink, affirm your release

Walk it off – Work it out, when in doubt. Let negativity and fear of being your true self flow. Overcome fear from your mind and heart with each step.

Reach out to your coach or guide and discuss your concerns.

Watch your thoughts and words. Keep your inner house clean. Be confident. Remember you can create anything you desire out of your vision.

Never forget that you deserve to live your purpose. When in doubt, fast your way through on nutrients, herbs and green vegetable drinks.

Write a gratitude letter in advance with your appreciation about bringing forth your vision.

Meditate.

Pray.

Affirm: *I am not afraid; I have complete trust in the birth of my vision work.*

Live fully from the Womb of Your Mind, the Womb of Your Heart and the Womb of Your Reproductive Center. Conceive your authentic self, come full term.

LABOR AND DELIVERY

Prepare your soul to experience a rebirth.

Ride the waves of the delivery process.

Relax & let go...

Nature is taking its course. You have come to the place of birthing your vision, your work. Fear not, it is time to bring your work to the world. In labor, your fears may heighten. Trust yourself. Breathe deeply. Push yourself through. Let go. You've done the necessary work to have a beautiful birth. Stay in prayer. As you keep on letting go, embrace yourself with only the strongest, most positive reflections to help open you up to your greatness.

Trust that you and your vision are going to be fine. Ride the birthing contractions, regardless of how intense they are. When you look back, you will reflect, that it was worth all that you went through to reach the illumination of your vision.

Congratulations! You've delivered your vision. The challenging labor is over. Your vision is here, you've done it. You are the victor. Check to see if your work is in tact. Count its toes and fingers and its spirit. Your vision has survived your inner journey. You endured, and thereby brought your vision into a reality. Now you must ready your soul for the next journey as your vision begins to grow.

Embrace the birth of your work, your life!

AFTER THE BIRTH

All is well. Your vision has been born. For a while your vision must remain very close to you for nourishment and care as you nurture your work, into maturity, strength, and power. Use your support team to assist you. Continue to embrace and love your vision.

Watch out for post-partum blues. Rest and reflect. Regain your balance (take hot baths, light a candle and meditate as you soak in and appreciate the birth.) To further avoid post partum blues, embrace the birth soulfully as you give thanks for it.

Suggested post-delivery activities:

- Through e-mail and/or land mail send out announcements for all to witness your newly arrived, via promotion, internet, radio, cable TV, newspaper, magazine.
- Have a community welcome.
- Present an "Open House".
- Have a release Party.
- Have a press party.
- Have a viewing.

YOUR VISION MATURES

Now that your vision is born and the world has received it, the greatest task is to continue supporting it to maturity. You want your vision to become well-established and to support you spiritually, physically and financially. If you become worn out or tired while growing your vision; or you run out of funding or faith, rest, reflect and recharge. Then get back on the road to success with everything you have within. In business, it usually takes at least 2 years (8 seasons) for your business to "take hold". Your work has then passed the test of time and has the potential to reach full maturity.

You must water and nurture your work daily. Do this through the constant promotion, advertisement, re-evaluation, and shaping of your work to connect to the needs of the people. Stay connected to the voice of the people, and their quest will help you to shape your vision into work that is both rewarding to you and relevant to the times. To maintain, keep your works in the eye of your community, and in the eye of the world. Continue to study and develop your crafts and skills in your field. Witness your vision grow as you develop yourself from the inside out.

Give thanks and celebrate!!!

I JUST WANNA TESTIFY

To heaven from hell-right here on earth…
I am here to testify that my womb has experienced a re-birth…
I am here to tell it, sing it, dance it, spell it…
However you want it. I just want you to hear it.
I am here to tell you that my womb has survived…
My womb has been resurrected from the darkness,
My womb has walked through the fire; and stood the tests of time,
My womb is no longer in the dark,
By way of fasting, cleansing, and prayer
My womb can stand up and say, "Don't you dare!"
To any man who dares to try to take away what's mine
By way of baths, herbal tonics, and more prayer,
My womb has come to see a grand and glorious day…
By letting go of meats that held sorrowful defeats,
My womb has been able to release,
Release the rape, the pain, and the horrors of trauma,
That has been brought to me by my father,
Release the betrayal, hurt, and confusion,
Brought to me by so many other men,
I release the blame, the shame, and the guilt
I held within,
Because my daughter…
By letting go of all the flesh that nearly brought death
I can finally feel the power of my breath
The power that has renewed my womb and being.
Yes, given my womb a brand new tune.
By cleansing and purging, I can now see
My womb was not meant to bleed seven days
I am now down to only three…
My womb is so great,
She is so free, She was re-invented
It almost seems.
She is so full of joy and laughter
She's just too hard to keep up after
She became filled with so much love and joy
She naturally birthed me an organic baby boy!
When the delivery was finished
She was so conscious
She did not even need a stitch
Just a little bit of olive oil did the trick
Oh yes, oh yes my womb has seen a new day,
She is so happy to be reborn
She has returned to her natural form
To heaven, from hell, right here on earth
I am here to testify
My womb has experienced a rebirth.

Sacred Woman Ta Mer Ra het-Heru
(La Tayla Monique Palmer-Lewis)

WOMB OVERLOAD; WOMB RECOVERED

My womb screamed. She shouted and hemorrhaged monthly. She endured many years of pain. I needed extreme measures to heal myself. As a "sun person", my womb "requests" pulled me towards a warm climate. So, I purchased two airplane tickets to St. Thomas in the US Virgin Islands for myself and my youngest son, Ali. I kissed and hugged everyone farewell and left on my quest to save my womb...and my life.

After six months under the tutelage of Mother Nature; after "surgery" through sun, air and sand baths and ocean salt-water soaks, my womb and I rose to exceptional heights. During this period I slowed down my living pace. I saw only those few clients who could find me up in the tropical hills delicately embraced by the Caribbean Sea. I got plenty of rest and spent energizing time with my sister and beloved friend, Dino Joseph, a powerful healer residing in St. Thomas who took Ali and me under her wings. Although, I had to leave my husband along with my other children in the States for that time, peace began to re-establish itself in my womb and my life. I began to reflect a newfound peace and serenity.

When the Caribbean environment had healed us, we gathered our strengthened beings and returned to New York. Ali was revitalized and finished the school semester. My womb healing journey had saved my life. My womb had been with me for four decades and deserved an honorable healing. It was a blessing to be able to give her the divine attention, time and sun-charged rest that she deserved. My womb had survived many trials and tribulations through my ignorance, my boyfriends, my husbands, my divorces, my hurts, my PMS, my chronic menstrual pain and excessively heavy menstrual flow. Together my womb and I fought the battle of Cesarean delivery (C- section) to bring my three beautiful children to earth.

I used to reflect on how the deliveries caused war scars to my womb. Of, course, when I reflect on my three children, (now adults) I realize they are the "Purple Heart" medals that I earned. Blissfully, from both my personal healing and my desire to help women to overcome their health and wellness challenges, I also "won" knowledge. Now I know that childbearing does not have to be a battle. There do not have to be war scars.

We're alive! My womb and I have survived to tell the story. I am able to be a guiding light of inspiration. I am able to encourage women and men to step forward and awaken their self-healing ability. I am living the wellness and restoration of my womb, my Seat of Creation.

I am delighted to share the wellness with you.

Queen Afua (1994, 2009)

Sacred Gathering of Wombmen Circle Testimony

SHARED THROUGH
ABU'T NBT MUT DR. CHENZIRA D. KAHINA KHERISHETAPHERU

Our center is where our wombniverse rests;

Each birth and rebirth of an idea, action, and work are...heavenly..."

–From Sacred Mother of Creations © 2000–Dr. ChenziRa D.K.K.herishetapheru

Every wombman's lotus transformational journey bears an individual embrace of our sacred elements of air, fire, earth, and water –A FEW womb charging qualities. As technological globalization consumes our earth and damages our environments, it is our charge as Womb Workers living in the highest heights to forge ahead with spiritual actions that will invoke the wombmanifestation of global healing to save humankind. This wombniversal healing vision serves as a paradigm for establishing, maintaining, and globalizing Womb Healing & Womb Wisdom Workers' circles for lotus transformation, our sacred reality.

Healing Circles exploded upward out of mud-like netting complimented by the Caribbean Sea that surrounds our tropical isle. Our wombmen came to receive revelations from our Mother Father of Creation as NTR. Share, learn, grow, be nurtured and fed from the oceans of healing space shared among our bodies, souls, and consciousnesses. Wombmen of our Caribbean community and abroad began to relearn and revisit their abilities to meditate, pray, sing, chant, dance, sew, plant, cry, and heal together. Every evening Nut graced us within the embracing womb of our Sacred Gathering of Wombmen Circle. Per Ankh reactivated lotus seeds for transformation that were dormant and lacking natural springs of water for a considerable time. The wombs of our women, men, and families have been awakened.

WOMB WORKERS AWAKENING

Calling on Womb Workers! Calling on Womb Workers!
As above so below.
As within so without.
The state of the earth; the womb of the elements of nature; and
The state of humanity reflects itself as womb unrest.
We are the Womb Workers and we activate.
We are the women who have lightened the darkness.

As we rise we end the low consciousness of humanity
That has created
As the Gatekeepers of humanity's entry onto planet earth
And Womb Workers of natural living
Through our thoughts, words & deeds
We have taken on the mantel to birth a New World
The ancestors of antiquity said,
"I speak that, I wish and it becomes strong,
It comes into existence as I speak."
As Womb Workers, we accelerate with great devotion
The healing principles of Womb Restoration,
We give birth to healthy thoughts
In order to breed Womb Restoration
The becoming of whole souls is our charge.
As a Womb-Wisdom Worker,
I assist women in sharing their stories
In a safe womb circle that womenfolk may
Individually and collectively
Purge and rejuvenate all our lives.
As a Womb Worker, I take responsibility
In wholistically healing my womb conditions
I will conceive healthy relations
With The Divine,
With my relationships, with nature
And with myself.

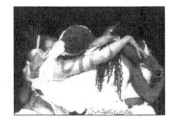

As a Womb Worker,
I actively spread wellness
Globally, for the betterment of humanity.
As a Womb Worker,
I am here to end world suffering
First, by sharing, guiding, learning with and teaching women,
To respect, honor, and purify themselves
that they would be reborn
as whole, beautiful and honorable.
I am a Womb Worker and I am here to birth a New World.
As a womb worker, I am here to share, learn with
Guide and to share with our men, from birth,
How to respect and purify themselves
That they may be reborn
As whole, beautiful and honorable men.

PORTAL

Five

CELEBRATION

There are 108 poses of the Womb Yoga Dance
designed to protect the reproduction center
by the joining of breath and movement.

To unify and harmonize,
both men and women are encouraged
to perform these movements.

CELEBRATE YOU

*Y*ou deserve to celebrate. You have weathered storms. You have listened to and lived stories. You have detoxed for restoration of wellness to your womb and your entire body. You are daring to rebirth yourself and your vision. You testify that some days are easy and some days the challenges for balance and wellness are overwhelming. Dear Ones, continue to drink your tonics with devoted efforts to heal thyself. Your prayers of thanksgiving and forgiveness are restoring the wombs of your hearts. You had the courage to admit you *might* have an angry vagina; you felt sad or afraid. You put the book down and said, "No, that's not me." Then you juiced some organic green vegetables and said, "This isn't *that* bad." When you took a hot bath with special oils that smell lovely, you thought, *"Mmmm, this feels sooooo good."* You memorized some affirmations. You are re-empowered; you make choices about what you will **eat** and **say** and **do** and *not* **do** for your own wellness. Recognize the blooming lotus that you are. Then, rejoice, **you deserve to celebrate.**

Dance of the Womb is a series of 39 movements. Womb Yoga is a series of 69 poses. Together these 108 movements and poses are the Womb Yoga Dance System of rejuvenation, tranquility and celebration. This system is a vaginal anitaging method of rejuvenation. Every movement in Dance of the Womb and pose in Womb Yoga has a message, a meaning and a purpose. They are meditations in motion. 108 is a number that symbolizes wholeness, completeness, creativity, enlightenment and transformation. Enjoy these states of wellness. Dance to continue overcoming an angry vagina and rebirthing your goals. Dance by yourself in front of the mirror. Push back the furniture and dance with your children, your mate and your parents. Dance for wellness. **You deserve to dance.**

Every culture has traditional dances that are passed from generation to generation. Celebrate the dances from your culture. All women and men, youth and elders are invited to perform daily, Dance of the Womb and Womb Yoga. Dance "Old School"; dance "New School". Use the poses presented here. Create your own steps and poses. As we heal ourselves, we heal our relations. Keep moving. Practice and perform these movements for wellness at your community and wellness centers and at retreats and reunions. Celebrate with the praise dances done in your house of worship. Help to raise the frequency of humanity and put an end to the hurt and angry wombs of the world. Collectively, we can overcome the catastrophic conditions that have plagued our earth and our bodies, minds and emotions. With dance, you can create an inner atmosphere of forgiveness and love. You can dance and begin to reflect tranquility and beauty from your insides to your outsides. Let Dance of the Womb and Womb Yoga be part of your glorious celebration of Wellness. **You deserve to move and to dance and to celebrate.**

WOMB YOGA DANCE SYSTEM
A WELLNESS MOVEMENT

Come, dance! Transform, yourself on the personal, global and cosmic levels.

Renew your womb centers; re-birth yourself and your work.

Usher new wellness into the human community.

Merge the Dance of the Womb (39 movements) with Womb Yoga (69 poses).

Connect to your Sacred Inner Geometry with these 108 movements.

Dance away disharmony and *dis*-ease; embrace harmony and wellness.

Breathe to align the wombs of your mind, your heart and your reproductive seat.

Dance and breathe these movements of a Womb Wellness Movement.

Rejuvenate through the forces of nature—air, fire, water, earth.

Dance upon your golden wings; breathe to soar to heights of wholeness.

Dance fully to spread a soothing wellness blanket over humanity.

Inhale deeply to bring oxygen and serenity into your womb center.

Exhale to release anxiety and tension from your life.

Raise your frequency with this powerful healing force.

Renew and rebirth your world; our world.

Come, dance! Womb Yoga Dance at the rising of the sun.

Come, dance! Womb Yoga Dance at the setting of the sun.

Dance to transform your spirit, body and mind.

Inhale Wellness through your breath, movements and thoughts.

Exhale the pain, the rage, the anger.

Visualize vibrant worldwide healing energy.

Forgive. Grow. Shine.

Dance and breathe to restore, love, beauty, balance.

Rebirth the Earth.

Celebrate a Womb Wellness Movement

Dance of the Womb

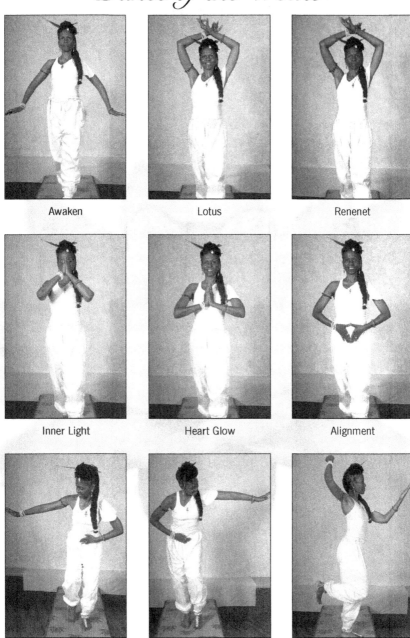

Awaken

Lotus

Renenet

Inner Light

Heart Glow

Alignment

Healers Unite (right)

Healers Unite (left)

Drum Call

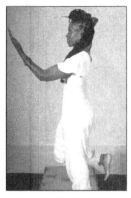

Four Corner Drum Call

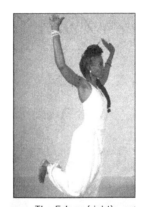

The Falcon (right)

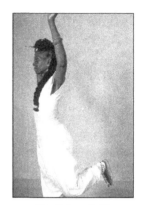

The Falcon (left)

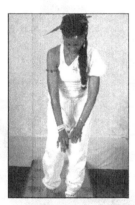

Planting Seeds

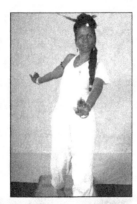

Planting Seeds Around the World

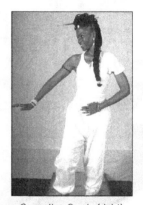

Spreading Seeds (right)

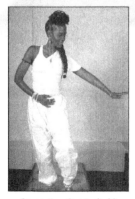

Spreading Seeds (left)

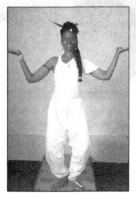

The Ancients

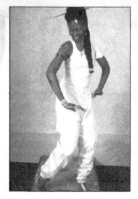

Go Within (right)

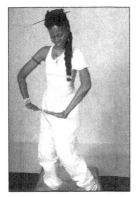

Go Within (left)

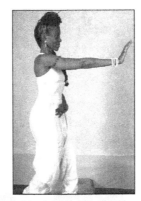

Womb Protection (right)

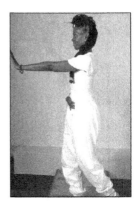

Womb Protection (left)

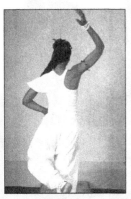

World Womb Wellness

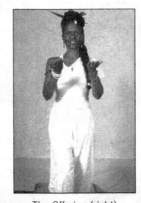

The Offering (right)

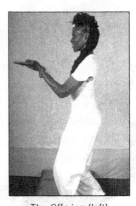

The Offering (left)

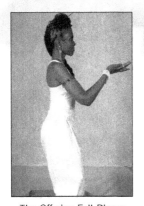

The Offering Full Bloom

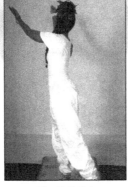

The Call Out

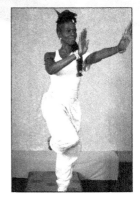

Global Rise

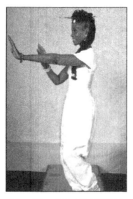

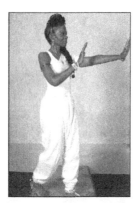

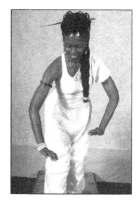

Four Directions Protection (right)

Four Directions Protection (left)

Stir the Herbal Pot

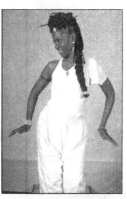

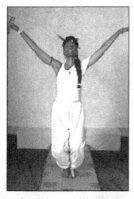

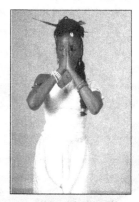

Womb Divine

World Womb Wellness

Womb Center

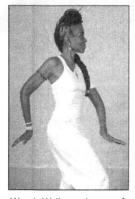

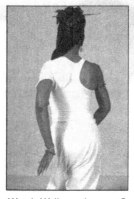

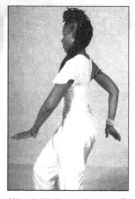

Womb Wellness Journey 1

Womb Wellness Journey 2

Womb Wellness Journey 3

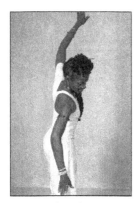
Falcon Soar

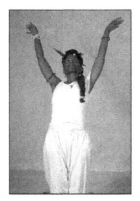
Womb Liberation

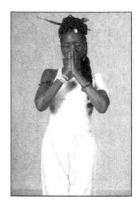
The Healer Within
Awakens

Womb Yoga

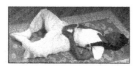
The Rebirthing Pose

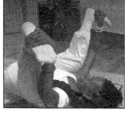
The Advanced Rebirthing
Pose

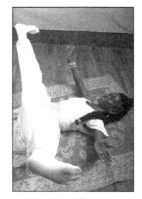
The Lotus Blossom

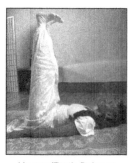

Heaven/Earth Balance

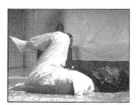

The Womb Seat

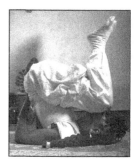

Inner Reflection

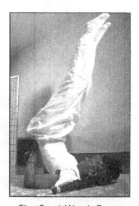

The Great Womb Purge

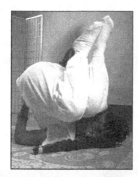

Inner Sanctum (left)

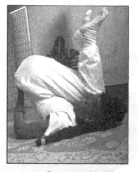

Inner Sanctum (right)

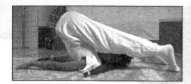

Advanced Inner Sanctum

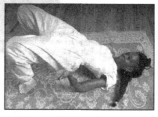

Advanced Bridge Over
Troubled Water

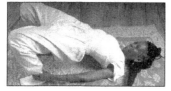

Bridge Over Troubled Water

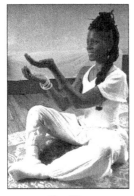

The Altar

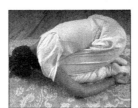

The Fetus

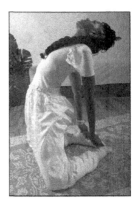

The Mountain

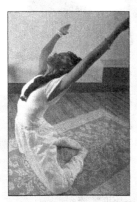

Sunburst

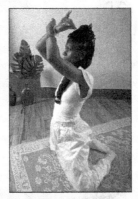

Lotus Blossom

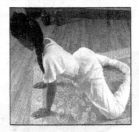

Waterfall

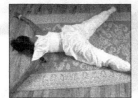

The Offering

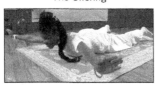

The Womb Lift

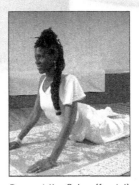

Renenet the Cobra (frontal)

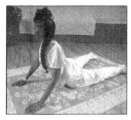

Renenet the Cobra (right)

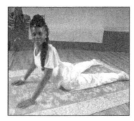

Renenet the Cobra (left)

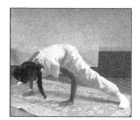

Meshkenet Birth

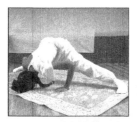

Meshkenet Adoration

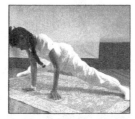

Empowered Meshkenet

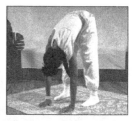

Wombniversal Nut

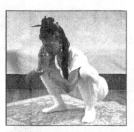

Ast Seat of Power

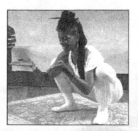

Womb Offering

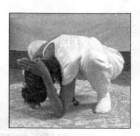

Cosmic Womb

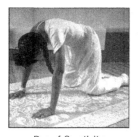

Bes of Creativity

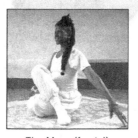

The Moon (frontal)

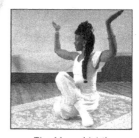

The Moon (right)

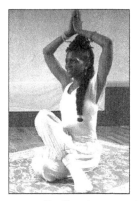

The Temple

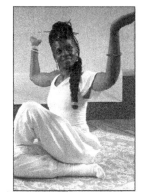

The Moon (left)

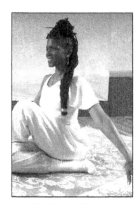

The Moon (frontal)

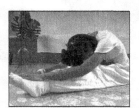

The River Flows

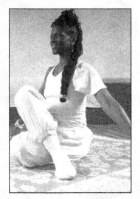

The Moon (frontal)

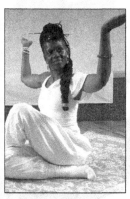

The Moon (left)

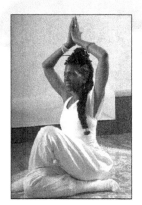

The Temple

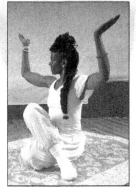

The Moon (right)

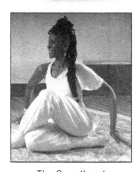

The Sweetheart

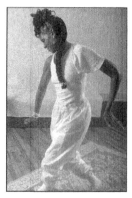

The Global Rise

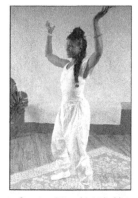

Sunrise Bliss (right/left)

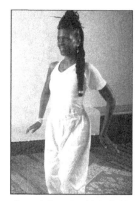

Sunset Serenity (right/left)

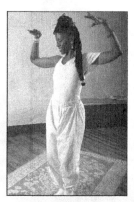

Renenet Wise Awakening

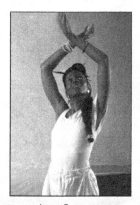

Love Supreme

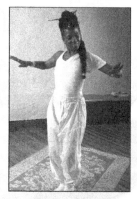

Seven Aritu Chakra
Balancing

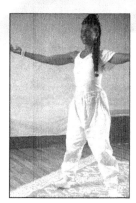

Four Direction Sacred
Geometry

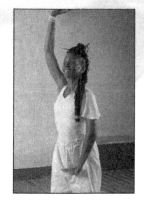

Four Direction
Heaven/Earth Union

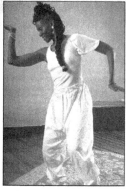

Time Traveler (right)

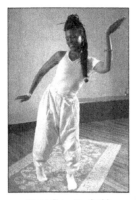
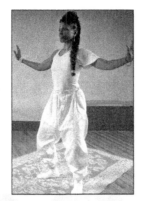
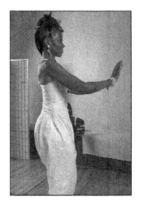

Time Traveler (left)   The Volcano   The Volcano Erupts
                           Opens(right/left)

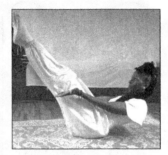

The Pyramid

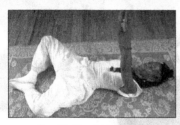
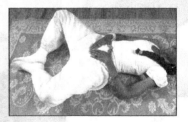

Sun Ra Pyramid Charge   Womb Rejuvenation

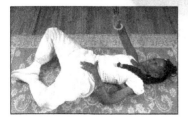
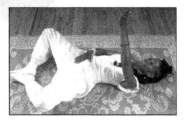

Renenet Womb Rejuvenation (right)   Renenet Womb Rejuvenation (left)

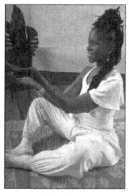

The Altar

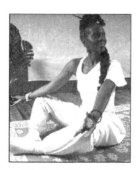

Womb Spinal Stretch

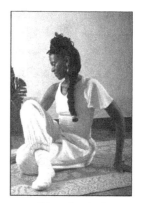

Falcon Perched

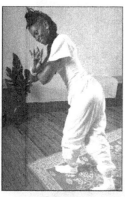

Falcon Rises

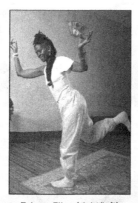

Falcon Flies (right/left)

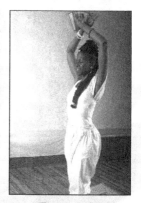

Temple Light

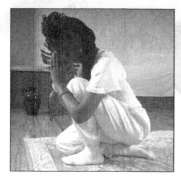

My Daily Womb Healing Prayer

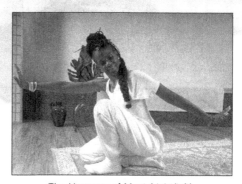

The Harmony of Maat (right/left)

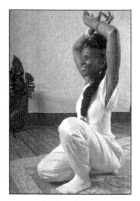 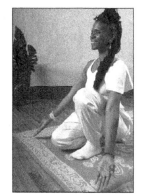

Sitting Lotus   New Beginning

WHOMB?

Delta mama with your fertile
Loins of lavish strength
Hammock to the generations
Of our babies nestled beneath the full moons of your breasts
I remember you rich resplendent wombman
With your "melanific" indigo hue
Your hips swaying
Sashaying pelvic mementos to a Congolese beat
Even the sweat from your brow tasted
Honeysuckle sweet
Oh, how life adored you
From your pyramidal third eye
To the soles of your butterscotch feet
Solomon's mines paled against your golden treasury
Egyptian cotton could not hide your incandescent beauty
Beloved, my beloved
In those beginnings, whomb of we could have ever seen
The decline of our power
The invasion and pillage of our sacred V's
This lotus flower now cursed it seems
To weather its' withering enslaved by
Submission to carnal creeds
Each womb of us carrying mangrove memories
Implanted deeper within us than our arms will ever reach
I have asked of midnight to give us back our dreams
I have asked thunder to silence the cacophony
Chorus of angered contractions held hostage
By swollen caustic screams
I have asked the voices in the waters
To help us heal this endless hemorrhaging

I ask
I implore
I beseech
For every thrust received against a wooden floor
For every garment torn asunder
For every knife that cut us all
For every razor edge and blunder
For every hand that muffled fear
For every statute cavalier
For every ounce of crimson blood
Spilled from our legs
Drawn from our veins
From every scalpel spliced solution
I call upon these tender folds of flesh
To claim itself as restitution
Now, body rise!
Wombward!
I ask of you
Whomb but we can overcome our angry V's
No longer victims
But architects of revolution
Whomb?
Yes
We

Faybiene Miranda
2/5/10

OVERCOMING

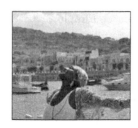

Global Women hands to the sky
Seek refuge in nature
Ask the rain to assist in the cleanse
And the winds to dust out unwanted clutter
Bathe in the glory of the sun
and drink water fresh from the stream
Rest under honeydew grass
whilst the morning birds sing sweet lullbies
on fruit laden trees
Beware of pretty distractons,
Stay focused on your journey
Let your spiritual compass show you the path to walk,
the bridges to cross
and the barriers to knock down.
Continue to dance as sunsets,
Let your belly rejoice in the warmth of the night
As moonlight whispers the truth of your great transformation.

By DD McCalla

THE 65-YEAR GESTATION

Mostly we women of a certain age wanted a different childhood, resulting in different teen years, a more sacred and admired adulthood.

Mostly we women of a certain age wanted encouragement to create, to glow, to prosper, to follow our most intangible dreams.

Mostly we women of a certain age wished for support, contentment with our bodies, self-admiration, self-sufficiency. We wished to be perfectly acceptable in our own skin.

Our cultural references, however, told us that we must be demure underpinnings of other people: diaper those babies, cook for that man, make a serene home for elderly parents.

Our jobs and careers could support others' successes: teachers, not principals; nurses, not doctors; bookkeepers, not CPAs; nuns or wives of pastors or rabbis, not spiritual leaders.

And so, following these preset conditions, I lived my life in a skin that fit me like someone else's.

All my life I yearned to be a singer. But I was discouraged vehemently; young women with solid plans for their futures could be nurses or teachers or maybe social workers, but nothing uncertain or frivolous, like entertainers.

I did not entertain anyone through my high school and college years, my teaching years, my married years, my parenting years. I did not perform when my husband died, when my son graduated from M.I.T., when my parents celebrated their 65th wedding anniversary. I did not collect paychecks for gigs either in bars or opera houses, only in schoolrooms. And always a yearning made my throat close before I could cry out for this singer inside my womb, waiting to emerge, waiting to be born.

Diagnosed with multiple sclerosis at age 58, I realized that I had gestated long enough; it was time to give birth to the singerwoman. This heresy, however, is antithetical to all training we women of a certain age had.

The "womb" is not only a biological term; it is also a concept: an internal sense of self, pregnant with possibilities and desires as well as fetuses. It is a place of comfort and security where something can be nurtured and protected. Sometimes those concepts and yearnings exist in our wombs for a very long gestation.

I needed to use my womb to give birth to my own self's reality. And, like physical pregnancies, although some may naturally abort, the strong ones flourish.

Labor is a long and arduous process that involves an ingathering of others in the universe to make a successful birth. Mine included 4 different voice teachers to give me different levels of courage to open my voice and soul, 2 different accompanists, and sisters to support me through self-doubt. Each risky step, scary and halting, required massive breaths through deliberate respiratory techniques.

The birth of the singerwoman was celebrated at the Metropolitan Room in New York City on Sunday, October 4 and Sunday, October 11 at 4 pm. She is 65 years old, 218 lbs, 5'7", with red and white hair and blue eyes. She sings out loud, and she will continue to sing. After all, it was what she was born to do.

Maxene Kupperman-Guiñals

Triumph

My mother said, "Keep your credit clean." My father said, "Pay your taxes and purchase the building that houses your work." The business owner says, "Get a loan." The wise one says, "Become a not-for-profit organization and get funded by other people's money, your community, or by large corporations." I did it the "old school" way: I relied on myself for funding; meaning I sold my products and services, and reinvested the profits to build my business: my sacred work. Over the years, it was very difficult to maintain. A fire on the premises, the flood that washed my business away and the padlock placed on my door by the city for unpaid rent, forced me to move my business. I was forced to move from one location to the next –eleven times! With the added expense caused by each move I still could not afford to buy the building as my father had suggested. I had to rent.

In 1993 my mother purchased the building I'm in now and put it in my name. Between the support of my mother's purchase and my husband's labor of reconstruction, my work stabilized immeasurably. It has been a wonderful, exciting, frightening, "make ya wanna holla", loving, and sacred journey. In the early days I had a staff of 7 that included 4 colon therapists, 2 masseuses and a secretary/manager. The location was in an affluent neighborhood and I had plenty of business and more clients than I could handle. This was the heyday of my work. However, due to my unsophisticated management skills (at that time), I had to close down my business abruptly. The city marshals came with padlocks in hand and gave me 30 minutes to pack up my children and my business and move out. After moving expenses, I was left with $30.00 and no source of an income. With no finances, how was I to take of my three children or my vision? I may have been short on money, but I was *never* short on creativity and faith. In those areas, I've always been abundantly wealthy. Creativity and faith is what ultimately brings me financial stability every time.

I invested the $30.00 into a bag of clay and some herbal extracts that enabled me to produce 12 jars an herbal infused clay mixture. One month after being escorted by the city out of the building that had housed my home and my business; I created a wellness seminar and sold all the jars of the first jars of Queen Afua Rejuvenating Clay. I had created the wellness seminar, too. I had no money to rent out space to present a seminar, so I sat down with a lovely and patient woman at the rental office of the Bed-Stuy Restoration Company. I explained to her my story and my desire to continue to serve the community. She supported my vision. She allowed me to pay for the space with my proceeds *after* my presentation. The presentation was a smashing success; the people came out hungry for the healing. After the presentation, I had enough money from the clay sales and the seminar to pay for the space and make a sizeable profit. Not only was I able to purchase food for my children and myself, but I also tripled my clay inventory. Within 6 months of consistent work I was able to rebuild my business. When I think back about the city locking me out of my living and working space, having to say good-bye to my devoted staff, being temporarily out of work and having to carry my children with me to my mother's, all I can say is, "Give thanks." Those challenges were the beginning of a new level of my work. It was then that I had time and space to write my first book and create my product line. The writing of *Heal Thyself for Health and Longevity* changed my life forever. It became the catalyst by which I reached out and assisted thousands world-wide to journey onto the path of Wholistic Wellness. It has allowed me to leave a healing legacy for my children's children, and for planet Earth. My triumph is the many stories I have lived; the hard times and the good times. Through them all I remain committed to living my vision. My vision and I are in a sacred union of love and devotion. Together we reach for the height that gives us wings and lets us fly.

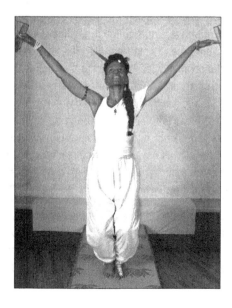

Celebrating Me

Use this space to put words, doodles and /or photos. Record your thoughts and actions of blooming into the lotus you are. Celebrate yourself.

Epilogue

"Women, come together as women healing on the last day of our fast in temples, shrines, churches, synagogues, mosques, day care centers, women shelters and in our homes to witness the atomic power of fasting and prayer through the honoring and the great purging of wombs everywhere. Cry for ourselves and each other and for what we, as women, bring to this earth. Let it be so, for this day we cry a river of tears that heal, so, that our strong tears wash this poisonous earth clean, and all of our sadness and despair will be washed away."

Upon finishing this statement, I dropped my forehead onto a mat on the wooden floor in my small writing room. I began to cry from inside. No tears rolled down my face because the cry was so deep. I had been channeled. I had given all of my energy. I embraced the reality that my Womb Wisdom was attempting to reach farther and farther.

At times during the process I felt sad and helpless, and at times helpful and so powerful. With my eyes full of uncried tears, I looked in the midst of my writing and there she was, Nut, the universal Sky Mother. She was crying too, and at that moment we bonded. I felt we were feeling the same, for in between her rain drops, my waters flowed. It was like the water that breaks when a womb opens to prepare for birthing. A revolutionary freedom movement was birthing itself on earth; I had tapped into every woman's wombstory.

Supa Nova, my eldest son, had been watching me work on this project for years, so he understood my many moods. In my state of melancholy, he handed me a green vegetable juice to drink. He said, "Drink this Ma, so you can be a stronger channel for your womb work." Holding the glass of juice seemed just too heavy as everything within me felt...gone. I was drained, but he insisted. I finally complied because I knew it was for my divine good. Supa Nova stood over me until I swallowed the last drop of juice. Then he began to jump and stomp in rhythm like a soldier. He put his fist up in the air and sang aloud, "Womb Power", "Womb Power", "Womb Power" until I got up off the floor and joined him in this *freedom dance.* We went on and on; we were charged and rejuvenated by our dance. We just danced and stomped and shouted, "Womb Power" all up and through the house. I picked up my drum and we were gone. It was like the whole world was ringing in harmony for the resurrection of the womb. We jumped, we swung, we swayed projecting and feeling and seeing and knowing Wombs were healing everywhere; birthing a New World through our prayers.

After our drumming, singing, shouting, and dancing we fell to the floor in laughter and joy. I thanked my son for being a seer, for picking me up from the floor and nourishing me with green juice and encouraging me to go on with the sharing of my womb vision. His participation helped to secure a wholistic and healthier future on earth for his children, for his contemporaries and for himself. I will forever think of those moments when I am in need of reassurance and I will give thanks and praise.

In the final channeling of **Overcoming,** I spent much time in my mother's garden looking out at her lilacs and sharing with my editor the words on these pages. I drank in the chlorophyll from the green fields and absorbed the warmth of the sun's rays. I watched the insects crawl and the butterflies in flight. I love what nature does to make us whole.

I am connecting to you; listening to your hearts' desires; paying attention to your cries to heal and overcome.

To have walked with you on this journey has been a gift of life... a love supreme.

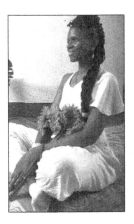

Dearest granddaughters
Maatia Torian and Atnnt Ne Neferáe Torain
This is for you, beloveds.

Love, Yaya

GLOSSARY

108 –
Number of positions and poses in the Womb Yoga Dance System

28-Day Global Womb Detox and Rejuvenation –
suggested plan for achieving global wellness

AIDS –
(Acquired immune deficiency syndrome) a disease of the human immune system

Balance –
stability; evenness

Bathhouse –
spa; place for using steam and sauna rooms; also for bathing and swimming

Bloodline –
family background; lineage

CENTER OF THE UNIVERSE –
metaphor for middle point of the whole

Clay –
earth; mud

Colon –
part of the intestine – vital to the digestive system for waste elimination

Common Ground –
literal term for place of mutual experience

Dance of the Womb –
a series of 39 movements designed for maintaining womb wellness

Detox –
(detoxification) - to cleanse from poisons, to purify

Elements –
basics; Ether, Air, Fire, Water, Earth

Enslavement –
condition of involuntary servitude

Essential Oils –
oils extracted from plants

Female Genital Cutting (FGC) –
controversially known as both female circumcision and mutilation

Gemstones –
minerals and stones

Global Epidemic –
plague or illness affecting people around the world

Herbs –
plants used for cooking and/or medicinal purposes

Hysterectomy –
partial or total surgical removal of the uterus

Imbalance –
unevenness; inequality

Ishe Oluwa Koleba Jeo –
(Yoruba) West African proverb: The Most High's work is indestructible and infinite.

Racism –
denial of rights and privileges based upon one's race

Rape –
crime of violence forcing unwanted sexual intercourse on someone

Rejuvenation –
restoration; renewal

Rite of Passage –
event or ceremony that marks transition from one stage of life to another

STDs –
sexually transmitted diseases

Toxic Lifestyle –
lifestyle that does not support wellness

Uterine Fibroids –
unwanted fibrous tissue growth on and around the uterus

Womb –
place of origin. A woman's uterus is the reproductive womb. Metorphorically, the heart is the "womb" of feelings and emotions; the mind is the "womb" of thoughts.

Womb Wellness Circle –
a gathering of women for sharing stories and rejuvenation

Womb Yoga –
a series of 69 poses designed for womb rejuvenation

Womb Yoga Dance System –
108 movements (39 Dance plus 69 Yoga) that join breath and movement for womb rejuvenation, tranquility and celebration.

Acknowledgements

MY ACKNOWLEDGEMENTS ARE MANY
AS ARE THE BLESSINGS THEY REPRESENT.

The concepts presented in *Overcoming an Angry Vagina: Journey to Womb Wellness* were first birthed nine years ago in the *Womb Worker Journal* and **The Womb Story** (a performance piece). **Special thanks to those original Womb Workers:** Conceptual Editor: Abu't Nbt Mut Ast Dr. ChenziRa D. Kahina-Kherishetapheru; (later) Literary Midwife/Editor; Kirsten Melvey; The Literary Womb Circle and cast: D.K. NeferAtum, Annette A-neith Irving, Auset Aswad, Ebony Ast Ra Kummba, Heathyre Mabin, Lady Prema, Mut Roseanne Ta-urt, Okera, Princess and her brother Don, Saraka. Also, the late, great Baba Kwame Ishangi, Sr., director, musician and actor. He is now enjoying his rightful seat as one of our ancestors.

Gratitude to the Womb Workers who supported my womb healing:
Mela Berger in Barbados whose healing hands charged my womb and Nicole Kruck of NY, who trained me in the Maya Womb Massage Technique and The Womb Spa founding practitioners: Fayola Herod, Fenenu McGee.

Gratitude for generosity of skills and talents:
Taziyah Naharah; "Thank you, for stabilizing "106" in Brooklyn."
SW Geodora Johnson-Bunn: "Thank you, for typing and driving and all you do."
Cheryl Audmond, Angie Bascom, Nzingha Evans, Lawanza Fewell, Domunique Hurd, Tanya Odums, SW Helen Walker, "Thank you for typing mountains of manuscript."
Autumn Marie, Mitzi Bryan: "Thank you for researching and editing manuscript each time I asked."
Cheryl Woodruff: "Thank you for the mercy and love that you extended to from your place inside the publishing world."

Gratitude and love to master publishers in London:
Ajani and Olayinka Bandele: "Thank you for publishing Overcoming and for distributing our wellness books and products in the UK."

Gratitude and love to new family of friends in London:
Mariandina Research Foundation - Stephen Ssali; Nubian Natural - Olayinka Bandele; Centerprise Trust Ltd. - Emmanuel Amevor; School of Unified Learning (SOUL) - Astehmari Batekun: A humble heartfelt Thank you to you and the London based community village radio station for your vibrant support. SW Nebt Tet for your commitment; SW Afiyo for your dedication; Ardela and Muntu of Emerald Arts: "Deepest Thank you." "Andy, you are a gem."

Humble gratitude for helping to birth the vision:
Nati and Afrakan World Press. "Thank you, for believing in and for publishing *Overcoming* in the US." Fredrica Bey, Wahida Mohammad, Roukiak Kamugisha, Osayande, Sonia Banner, Erykah Badu: "Thank you, all, for your financial generosity to help birth the wellness vision."

Profound appreciation:
Tony Fairweather: "Thank you, for launching *Overcoming an Angry Vagina: Journey to Womb Wellness* at the Celebration of Sistahs in London."
Les Brown: "For supporting my one woman show in the US."
Dr. Akua Gray: "You are a master administrator; thank you, for invaluable assistance in keeping our wellness work moving forward."
Dee Mc Calla: "Thank you, for your powerhouse skills of editing and for marketing our vision in London. You are Yum-licious!"

Great appreciation:
Jeff Shaw, Cindy Shaw and Camden Leeds: "Thank you for your support, your inspired talents for designs and lay-out for the book and mostly, for your generous patience."

Blessed Appreciation:
Joan Roper Adams, Chotsani Sackey: "Thank you, for reading and rereading."
Maxene Kupperman-Guiñals "Thank you, for being an extra pair of eyes."
Phyllis King-Robert, Yaani King, Zulliete Sanchez, Kelyse Marie Grant (age 9), "Grand Mary" Scott (Gerianne's mom), Ida Robinson (my mom): "Sisters, daughters, mothers, nieces, thank you, for the big things and especially for the little things."

Heartfelt appreciation:
"Big sister", Diana Pharr: "Thank you for your "on point" spiritual clarity and for knowing the birth date of *Overcoming*."
"My sister from another mother", Dr. Bernadette Sheridan: "I appreciate that through your master medical expertise and my wholistic conviction we share a vision of wellness for our community."

Great appreciation: To all the Women and Men who shared their stories.

Eternal gratitude: Hru Sen-Ur Ankh Ra Semahj Sa Ptah: "You are a royal King of Kings."

Profound gratitude: To the children of my physical womb—Supa Nova Slom, Sherease and Ali; and the child of my spiritual womb—Ka-mena. "Thank you for your continuous support."

Finally, Sister-girl Gratitude: For the big heart of Midnight Literary Midwife, Gerianne Francis Scott for her brilliant mind and tenacious, Taurus devotion to her work as Conceptual Editor of this text. "Woman, you have walked this literary road with me since *Heal Thyself.* I could not *have done birthed* this text without your loving support. Yes, now we can go dance at the beach."

Bibliography

Afua, Queen. *Heal Thyself for Health and Longevity.* New York: A&B Book Publishers, 1994.

Afua, Queen. *Sacred Woman: A Guide to Healing the Feminine Body, Mind & Spirit.* New York: Ballentine Books/One World/Random House. 2000.

Afua, Queen. *Womb Wisdom: A 28 Day Birthing Process Towards Global Healing.* 2009.

Dale, Cyndi. *The Subtle Body: An Encyclopedia of Your Energetic Anatomy.* Boulder, CO (United States): Sounds True, Inc., 2009.

compiled by Essential Science Publishing. Fourth Edition. *Essential Oils Desk Reference.* USA. 2007

Lark, Susan M., MD. *Fibroid Tumor and Endometriosis Self Help Book.* Berkley, CA. 1993, 1995, 2000.

Mendelsohn, Robert S., MD. *Male Practice: How Doctors Manipulate Women.* US. 1981.

Parvati, Jeannine. *Hygeia: A Woman's Herbal.* Albion, Calif: Freestone Publishing Company. 1978.

Pookrum, Jewel, MD. *The Medina Affect.* (audiotape). US. 1990.

Queen Afua's
Wellness Products & Services

Formulas

Heal Thyself Green Life Nutritional Formula I $24.00
Provides added nutrition to rejuvenate womb with nature's green whole
food supplements. Ingredients: Spirulina, Wheat Grass, Lecithin, Psyllium Husk

Heal Thyself Master Herbal Detox Formula II $24.00
To assist in detoxing the entire anatomy. Ingredients: Gota Kola, Pau D'Arco,
Alfalfa, Echinacea, Red Clover, Cascara Sagrada, Mullein, Chickweed,
Dandelion, Ginger, Parsley, Fenugreek, Blessed Thistle

Heal Thyself Inner Ease Colon Formula III $14.00
Aids in flushing the colon to relieve pressure from the womb.
Ingredients: Cold Pressed Olive Oil, Castor Oil, Vitamin E.

Heal Thyself Herbal Laxative Formula IV $12.00
Stimulates gentle colon cleansing for colon and womb wellness.
Ingredients: Cascara Sagrada

Heal Thyself Rejuvenation Clay Formula V (8oz.) $24.00

Heal Thyself Rejuvenation Clay Formula V (4oz.) $16.00
A body food for the womb containing supplemental zinc, calcium,
potassium, and magnesium. Ingredients: Green Clay, Red Clover,
Eucalyptus Oil, Peppermint Oil, Distilled water

Heal Thyself Breath of Life Formula VI $18.00
Helps open up and relaxes womb centers.
Ingredients: Pure Peppermint Oil and Eucalyptus Oil

Womb Aid Herbal Formula VII $18.00
A Womb Aid to rejuvenate & detox the womb with herbs from
nature's garden. Ingredients: Red Raspberry, Golden Rod,
Blue Cohosh, Don Quai, Dandelion, Red Clover

Womb Aid Clay Wonder Formula VIII $24.00
Helps soften & detox the womb. Black Earth, Bentonite Clay, Seaweed

Womb Aid Massage Oil Formula IX $15.00
Helps support womb circulation. Almond Oil, Flaxseed Oil, Olive Oil

Womb Wellness Products

Womb Wellness CD $20.00
Guidance for maintaining a vibrant, healthy womb.

Womb Heart Rose Quart Bracelet for Love and Forgiveness $12.00

Womb Heart Rose Oil for Womb Heart Balancing $15.00

Wellness Charts

All Charts $12.00

Womb Wellness Chart •• Nutrition Kitchen Chart •• The Liberation Pyramids of
Wellness Chart •• The Hydrotherapy Bathroom for Personal Wellness Chart •• The 7
Arit/Chakras for the Inner City of Wellness Chart •• The Road Map to Optimal Wellness
Chart •• Womb Yoga/Dance of the Womb Rejuvenation Chart •• Womb Wellness Chart

Wellness Consultations

1 hour . . . .$125.00/$185.00

Wellness Lifestyle Consultation One on One Session:
to Learn How Gain Optimal Wellness

Womb Spa Treatment $125.00

Wellness Certifications and Workshops

Emerald Green Practitioner Training $750.00

5 Day Training (Men and Women)

Overcoming an Angry Vagina:

Womb Wellness Lifestyle Practitioner Certification $495.00

3 Day Certification Training

Womb Yoga Dance Teacher Certification $455.00

3 Day Certification Training

Journey to Womb Wellness Certification $595.00

3 Day Retreat

Womb Yoga Dance Class . . . .$ 15.00

90 minutes

Women's Healing Soul Sweat . . . .$ 45.00

3 hours

Books

Heal Thyself: For Health & Longevity

Sacred Woman: A Guide to Healing the Feminine Mind, Body, & Spirit
The City of Wellness: Restoring Your Health Through the Kitchens of Consciousness

Wellness CDs

Wellness Lifestyle Consultation on CD $20.00/each

Family Package (includes 12 CDs) $179.00

Topics include: 21 Day Road Map for Optimal Wellness, Womb Wellness,
Prostate Wellness, Colon Wellness and more...

Call Now for FREE consultation of Products, Services & Programs
718-221-4325